Cancer, I'll Give You One Year

A Non-Informative Guide to Breast Cancer

*A Writer's Memoir,
in Almost Real Time*

Cancer, I'll Give You One Year

A Non-Informative Guide to Breast Cancer

A Writer's Memoir,
in Almost Real Time

By
Jennifer Spiegel

RESOURCE *Publications* • Eugene, Oregon

CANCER, I'LL GIVE YOU ONE YEAR
A Non-Informative Guide to Breast Cancer: A Writer's Memoir, in Almost Real Time

Resource Publications
An Imprint of Wipf and Stock Publishers
199 W. 8th Ave., Suite 3
Eugene, OR 97401

www.wipfandstock.com

PAPERBACK ISBN: 978-1-7252-5590-6
HARDCOVER ISBN: 978-1-7252-5591-3
EBOOK ISBN: 978-1-7252-5592-0

Manufactured in the U.S.A.   01/06/20

For Wendy, Melody, and Tim.

This is the book on marriage that Tim and I will never write together.

I sometimes think one writes to find God in every sentence. But God (the ironist) always lives in the next sentence.

—"I Am Writing Blindly" by Roger Rosenblatt
in *TIME*, November 6, 2000

If I were a prisoner in Alcatraz, I'd be good so that I could earn privileges and have an accordion or something in my cell.

—Melody, June 2019

Preface

I originally wrote this as a private blog, in real-time, shared with a small group of interested—or supportive, at least—readers. *As things happened.* I've tried to remain faithful to that. I cut massive chunks, but I didn't change much or embellish conversations. I merely cleaned it up.

Initially, I had a long and unwieldy title that I still love: *Cancer, I'll Give You One Year: A Non-Informative Guide to Breast Cancer* Or *How to Get Your Ba-Da-Bing Boobies on the House!* The Ba-Da-Bing is a strip club in HBO's *The Sopranos.*

As you read, please do not forget the "Ba-Da-Bing" part.

Jennifer
October 2019

1

Call Me Ishmael

An Introduction (Summer 2015)

This is a book about writing.

I've debated with myself over how much to tell, how much to hide. I don't want people to stare at my breasts, to contemplate their shape and size. I don't want pity. Most of all, I don't want the identity. I don't want it to take over. Who am I, after all? A woman? A wife? A mother? A creature? A person dying?

I'm a writer, I'm a writer, I'm a writer, I keep insisting.

And insisting.

The lady doth protest too much, methinks?

"I'm just another writer / still trapped within my truth," sang Dan Hill in "Sometimes When We Touch" from 1977—"A hesitant prize-fighter / still trapped within my youth."

At seven, when I first heard that, I knew: I was Just Another Writer Trapped Within My Truth.

This was my first assertion of personal identity.

Can you even imagine?

I Yam What I Yam, according to Popeye the Sailor Man.

But now: Am I too old for this shit? Should I just succumb to the newness, be like liquid that takes on the shape of its container, change color to suit my surroundings?

Is this, then, my new identity: cancerous, stricken, dying?

Rod Stewart once sang, "You wear it well."

I wear "stricken" well, I guess. My friends have always given that little side-glance wink to each other when they've seen me bubble over with enthusiasm at some zombie crap. I'm attracted to "stricken." Stricken flesh turned living dead. I'm drawn to the zombie narrative. "Stricken" may be my secret second nature.

Tim—my husband, my unlikely and tempestuous best friend—instantly balked at signs of my preoccupation with identity. In the beginning of our marriage, I'll bet he said, "Who do you think you are?"

That sounds like him, during those first few years.

He no longer asks it like this. It took us some time, but we finally settled into happy marriage. Now, he asks—a tad playfully—"Are you still on that thing?"

I'm contemplative now, under this disease paradigm, *that thing*: Is my identity with which I'm so concerned something I choose, I construct, or I am given?

Sometimes, I'm all defensive: *I'm a writer, no matter what you say.*

Sometimes, I'm in charge. *I picked writer, and there's nothing you or anyone else can do about it.*

Sometimes, others are in charge. *Don't make me write about this disease. Don't make me do it, damn you.*

Is identity so malleable? So dependent on circumstances and context? Must my identity be validated by other people to really be mine?

In other words, what determines who we are?

When I told Tim that my identity was at stake with this cancer thing, he dryly declared, "As always, your identity crisis has to do with your writing."

Which is to say: *How the fuck much longer are we going to go through this? Until I drop dead, my love. Until I'm fucking dead.*

But now we're adding my physicality (disease) to this identity equation, which has always been problematic for me (I mean, Sybil, the main character in my book *Love Slave*, has an eating disorder).

After all these years, I knew a few things about myself.

I knew, at least, I was a writer with boobs.

I HAD BOOBS.

My identity, for seemingly the billionth time, is in flux again.

Don't I get a choice here?

Must I embrace this cancer thing? Weave disease into my soul, turn it into prose—my own spun gold, a byproduct of a Rumpelstiltskin Affair? Extramarital, incidentally.

I don't want to be a cancer writer.

I want to write about other stuff.

Love, for instance.

I want to write about love.

I don't want to be the one who writes all about surviving cancer, or surviving cancer till I eventually die from cancer. I don't want to write about how I started eating healthy and I took control of my future and I stopped trusting doctors and went paleo or vegan or whatever-the-hell.

That is not the kind of writer I want to be.

So with this paranoia surrounding personal identity, am I acknowledging some weakness in me, some vulnerability to public opinion?

I think I am.

Yes, of course, cancer is now part of me, never to be ignored, but—fluid, constructed, bestowed upon—I see my own writerly palette, my own identity as writer, as larger than this crazy disease, which, like a kind of black smoke monster (à la *Lost*), wants to take up the whole of me.

Maybe that is where a plea resides: *Let my writerly palette be larger than this.*

I want to write about humans doing human things.

Sadly, humans get cancer.

There is a plethora of books on my table, our new ad hoc disease control center: *How to Tell Your Kids You May Die, What to Eat Now That You May Die, How to Love Your Spouse Now That He or She May Die, Five Million Things to Do Before You'll Probably Die.* I haven't picked up any of them.

I submit my body. I submit.

Not so my personal identity. It's still mine.

And here we go: I write.

Damn it, I write.

2

Shake It Out (July 1, 2015)

I was diagnosed with breast cancer on Tuesday, June 30, 2015, around 2 p.m.

I began writing that evening by 6 p.m.: *after* Tim rushed home from work as a chemist (picture him ripping off his white lab coat, removing goggles if he actually wears goggles, leaving work without telling a soul—he cried in the car all the way home), *after* the confused kids ended their fun (the gravity of my situation incommunicable to children), *after* I had to call the mom of my daughter's friend to pick the friend up from the failed playdate which would never be rescheduled (the mom was kind and quiet, accommodating, unquestioning), *after* Tim and I showed up at my OB/GYN unannounced and asked to see the doctor in person immediately because he needed to explain this; he needed to tell us how this happened; he needed to tell us how he *let* this happen.

To me.

This sounds like Day One.

A friend posted Florence and the Machine's "Shake It Out" on my Facebook wall. Isn't that what I do when I write?

How do I shake this one out?

Day One: will you allow for rambling, for a metastasis of thought?

It's always darkest before the dawn.

At this point, I have no clue what stage it is, if I'm going to die, if I'll have one or both breasts cut off, or if nothing will be removed at all. I will tell you this: I instantly feel that my body is my enemy.

My body is the enemy.

Shake it out.

Suddenly, unprecedentedly, I have an affection—*I'm not joking*—for Angelina Jolie, who preemptively got rid of the two cancer culprits. *Hero* seems like an OK word now. About this heroism, though. My initial impression is that when people speak out or go public about disease, heroism has very little to do with it.

I'll personally tell people anything. I've done obnoxious self-promo for my books that's proven costly. I like to divulge my own shit—because I see candor and intimacy as especially key in my own writing aesthetic (thank you, David Sedaris).

But you know what? I don't care about being heroic or courageous.

Mostly, if not exclusively, I just want my kids to be OK.

Not exclusively—that's a lie. I want Tim to be OK, as well. There are others. I feel horrible that my mom has to go through this. She's had a lot of loss in her life.

How heroic is that?

Or is it merely ordinary?

Shake it out.

I'm not afraid of death. I believe in God. I believe in life after death. I'll just go all Chris Pratt for a moment. Some of my writer friends are staring into this black hole of meaninglessness and trying to make sense of their lives—and I'm not there. I am very upset that my kids may suffer.

But I'm OK.

Shake it out.

Even though I just professed Chris Prattness, I should tell you: Cynicism is my first inclination. I'm all, *Oh, Wow, So I'm Going to Die.*

My husband has told me, "You need to get rid of that darkness."

After the first half-hour post-diagnosis, I wanted to discuss a plan for the kids: how to talk about my death with them, whether he would feed the kids that black stuff in the back of the refrigerator, who their current teachers are and where he's supposed to pick them up at school. And Tim wanted to talk about *fighting cancer.*

But I was, like, "Why? If I'm going to die, I'm going to die."

And why do I need a positive attitude? Do you really think that there are curative properties in a faux sense of victory over a disease that shows no mercy?

Is this my own black hole of meaninglessness?

Shake it out.

My children, my children: What about my babies? That's what I need to know.

Shake it out.

I believe in story, in narrative arc, in beginnings and endings. How will my story end?

Shake it out.

And what if I have lived the life I was meant to live? What if I have accomplished what I was meant to accomplish? What if this is my end?

Shake it out.

I know people don't want to hear this.

Tim doesn't want to hear it.

So this is a book about writing. For a long time, in various places, I've insisted on the need for redemptive endings, for closure. These are not happy endings; these are meaningful endings.

Maybe this is mine, my redemptive ending.

Right now, should I die, I'm not the person I wanted to be. This current incarnation reeks of failure. But there are parts of my life that have been properly, maybe fully, resolved.

Tim: We're (ironically?) in the process of selling our first and only home together (I got a call from Stanley Steamer about cleaning my carpets in the old house while on the table getting biopsied—I will remember this always, me on my back, the screen with the glowy scanned image of my breast and its lumps, my phone ringing, the medical person waiting, the "This will only take a minute" part). It's been a constant trip down Memory Lane as our home together is packaged, tossed, obliterated, transformed. All the My Little Pony merchandise, gone. My U2 posters, already in the new closet. Should we finally get new towels that don't smell faintly of mold? Our Memory Lane, our road, was rather rocky. Like crazy rocky. I mean, the first eight years were killer. Amazingly, we survived. Knees more than scraped, but limbs intact.

We are scarred, though; *do not look too closely at our naked flesh.*

And now, now, this?

We survived for me to die?

What if the purpose of my life—like, *The Purpose of My Whole Life*—was so that Tim might emerge on the other side of our rocky road, now equipped for the hard work of being a single dad—my own emergence beside the point?

Is that too awful to say?

Too horrible to believe?

Isn't it a redemptive ending?

Isn't it a perfect ending?

Doesn't it coincide perfectly with my self-professed writing aesthetic: Make art of oneself, embrace candor?

Maybe this is my moment, my death scene. I am another kind of Juliet.

My own life aspirations have always been simple: I've just wanted to be in love like some dumbass girl in a whirlwind romance, and I've always wanted to be a writer. Kids included. To be honest, I got those things! Yeah, they're not all that they're cracked up to be, but so be it.

Tim doesn't want me to say this aloud, to succumb. He wants me to have a positive attitude. He has asked, "Didn't you picture us growing old together?"

Yes, I did.

Wait. Did I?

Or did I just want it to be so?

That all said—all that I just said—*I will cut off my breasts, if that's what it takes.*

Shake it out.

Look, it's Day One.

I'll fight, OK?

For my kids. They're the ones, you know?

My children, my children: What about my babies?

Please, dear God, take care of my babies.

And, Tim, you be the fighter. You get through this.

Shake it out.

3

But I Will Tell You More (July 13, 2015)

Lean in.

In 2013, due to money, I stepped down from teaching college to try my hand at teaching middle and high school at a small private school. I had to stop saying *fuck* (they made me!), I had to justify my decision to teach James Baldwin (James Baldwin!) due to its risqué content, and I had to wear nylons more than I would ever care to. I also had to stop being a writer—because, well, my stuff is inappropriate for kids. I had to smother the part of my identity that felt the most authentic.

Identity crisis! Same old, same old.

Tim liked the money.

I liked the money.

I barely made anything, but it was more than I had ever made before.

We felt rich. Sometimes, we ate Egg McMuffins! We went to Disneyland!

I'm not joking. We went to Disneyland over parent-teacher conferences. I bowed out, citing previous arrangements.

We can set up a meeting some other time!

I made feeble attempts at working on my novel during this year. I blogged quite a bit, which created the illusion that I was still in the "game." (I was actually kindly reprimanded for my blog at one point, because it contained my semi-notorious cussing.) My laurels had always been minimal, so I couldn't really rest on them.

It didn't work out.

Actually, I sucked.

Like, I was the *Worst Teacher Ever.*

(I might also mention that I was unhappy.)

But I couldn't talk about it. My writing life was verboten.

So, one year later, I rushed back to the college classroom, where I could say *fuck* and teach James Baldwin.

Then this: Cancer!

Really?

Can't I have a little breathing space first?

For now, I tell you this: *I'm no survivor. I just write.*

And now I will speak to the ladies.

Women, this is how it happened: I found what felt like two lumps—but turned out to be three—in my right breast on a normal Friday night after the kids had gone to bed.

I was not doing any self-exam in the shower, erotically soaped up like a porn star in steam. I think we were watching TV. We must have been heading towards the "zone," clad in the unsexy garb of the sleepy and the married. (Were we watching *The Sopranos*? Yes, we were watching *The Sopranos*.) The couch was brown, an L-shaped sofa—too big for the room. (I seriously bought furniture that didn't fit our house, and I *kept* it.) I felt something, maybe one week after a routine OB/GYN exam in which nothing was detected. (The doctor had said something, though, that I will forever remember: "I pray every morning not to miss the breast cancer that one in eight women will get." He missed mine. *I was the one in eight.*) But now—Tony Soprano about to do business at the Ba-Da-Bing—I felt it in my right breast: a stone, a swelling, a cherry pit.

I went for a mammogram and ultrasound on that Monday. Two biopsies followed on the following Friday. I was diagnosed with cancer in one breast twelve days after that initial discovery.

Cancer comes to you: It comes without ceremony.

There are things you might want to know. I'm forty-five, and breast cancer isn't a part of my family history. My kids are little. I was working, haphazardly, on what would become *And So We Die, Having First Slept*. We had just moved into a new house. A trip to Disney World—Disney World!—was planned for late July with my husband's entire immediate family (Disneyland in 2014, Disney World in 2015!). My marriage was in good shape.

I don't know what I would've done otherwise—if my kids were older, if my marriage sucked. Would I have been more conservative in my approach, less drastic? How would my decisions be shaped by circumstances?

I am forever bewitched by these questions: How does one thing influence another? If this, then what?

I only made it to two doctor appointments after diagnosis, though I had multiple scheduled. (I had scheduled some in the car on the way home from my OB/GYN on that first day—right there, sitting shotgun next to Tim.) Apparently, one is supposed to shop around for professionals, take one's time, weigh one's options. One breast, two breasts, reconstruction on the operating table or no?

But my criteria for placing the knife in hand was different: *Who would do it first? Who could cut them both off as soon as possible?*

I wanted the cancer gone.

Who could do it first?

That's all I really wanted to know.

And so we launched, immediately, our search for a doctor who would cut them off as soon as possible.

I began with a recommended doctor. A woman. I should go with a woman, yes?

Tim fondly called her a *boobologist.* "She is all about the boob."

Her office was feminine, soft, pink and salmon, maybe powder blue (I don't really remember). Her furniture and lamps and end tables were like *The Golden Girls* or *Designing Women* props. Was that a painting of an ocean shore or a conch shell, or was it a Georgia O'Keeffe? A great big peachy vagina?

This doctor only did breast stuff—no general surgery. And when she examined me, she closed her eyes, almost meditating. The Zen of the Breast. Expert fingers pit-patted around my old flesh, my saggy boob.

Here today, gone tomorrow.

She didn't mince words. "A single mastectomy is called for."

We were not talking about a lumpectomy.

But I knew that I wanted a double mastectomy. I knew this right away. I had two babies, and I'd cut off my breasts so I could stay alive for them. "I need a double," I said.

A double-double.

I have always been like this: *When the shit hits the fan, I get down to business.*

"A double is your choice," the boobologist agreed. "We could schedule you after your trip to Disney World." Statistically, it was fine to wait, she insisted. People wait all the time (teachers wait for Christmas break, even summertime). "I couldn't operate before then, anyways." The Zen Master was going on vacation, too! A double mastectomy at the beginning of August! "Go on your trip," she said. "Have a good time!"

Have a good time?

Was that even possible?

There could be no good times.

But I liked her. I'd recommend her. I have nothing bad to say about her, except that I needed to cut off both breasts immediately and she wasn't available right away and I couldn't wait because I had cancer growing in my body and they didn't know if it was spreading and they wouldn't know until they got in there and tested lymph nodes in my armpit, but—in the meantime—the cancer could potentially be slipping through to other parts of my body, if it hadn't already done so.

Of course my husband's mother, my husband's father, my husband's brother, my husband's sister, my husband's brother's wife, the five small cousins, my husband, and my own two children were holding their collective breath in their respective states (Massachusetts, Oklahoma, and Arizona) for what became—I was given this one small thing—*my decision*: Would I cancel Disney?

Could I do the surgery after the trip?

If I got operated on, like, tomorrow, would I still be able to go to Disney World?

I knew I couldn't wait for surgery.

I knew I wouldn't wait surgery.

I knew before I said a word.

There was no way in hell I would be going to Disney World with boobs.

Tim liked that doctor; he liked her boob-centricity. So boob-a-licious. So Zen-y. "We should go with her," he said in the car. "She's good."

Ommmmmmm.

But we still went to see the second doctor that same afternoon.

"A single mastectomy is needed; a double is what many women your age opt for. Disney could come first, no problem." That's what the second doctor said.

Why the fuck did they all want me to go to Disney World so much?

This doctor was a general surgeon. A man. I did no research whatsoever. None. I guessed a few things: older but not that old, probably Jewish, likely a New Yorker.

"I could do it next week," he said.

Bingo!

Back in the car, Tim said, "I liked the first doctor better."

And I said, "We're going with the second one."

"You just want the Jewish New Yorker."

"I just want to get the cancer out as soon as possible."

But the Jewish New Yorker thing didn't hurt, either.

So I had a double mastectomy, friends.

11

Cancer, I'll Give You One Year

Last Wednesday, on July 8, 2015.
Boobs gone.

* * *

If you're keeping track of the numbers, the time elapsed between feeling lumps and cutting off both breasts was twenty days. Plain, simple, surgical.

There were other issues. The biggie: reconstruction.

I didn't know this going into this hellhole, but reconstruction is covered by insurance. We're talking fake boobs.

They'll give you fake boobs for free!

They surgically stick these things in you called "Tissue Expanders"— hopefully at the time of the mastectomy but sometimes later—which stretch your skin gradually like a balloon, and eventually are removed (surgically again) and replaced with permanent implants. How long it takes depends on how big you want them and how often you get them filled. (One goes in for appointments to fill them up gradually. It hurts for a while like getting one's braces tightened at the orthodontist, except these are one's fake boobs sewed onto one's now ripped-up chest.)

In the days between diagnosis and surgery—those frantic twenty days— I saw things.

One breast cancer survivor showed me her unreconstructed chest. I'll tell you what it's like: smooth, un-nippled, the rib cage faintly visible. Mildly alien. Jarring, but not grotesque. The sight was reassuring. *I could do this,* I thought. *This is something I could do.*

I also saw reconstructed breasts. A friend showed me hers. An acquaintance until the moment when she lifted her blouse to reveal her C+ implants, and we became close friends. *Bosom buddies!* I saw them, and, OK, I gasped. They looked awesome! *Hubba-hubba!*

So, how should I do this? Stay flat, translucent, extraterrestrial? Pump it up? Skip Disney? Go anyways? Do it later? This was my decision?

How badly did I want fake boobs?

I surprised myself, folks.

I would've thought I'd be one of those gals who didn't care, who accepted her flatness and reveled in her winning personality.

Instead, I got this pretty Top-Notch Plastic Surgeon, and we started the process on the operating table—which means that while the Jewish New Yorker was cutting them off, the Top-Notch Plastic Surgeon was inserting tissue-expanders into my flat chest to be gradually filled in a process that would take months and hurt more than the double mastectomy.

I must be a hypocrite.

What is it with me?

Remember my personal identity spiel?

Wasn't I above this hapless clamoring for physical beauty?

Why do women desire breasts?

What makes them so important?

And what do plastic surgeons tell their children they do for a living?

Can they sleep at night?

Twenty days after discovering lumps, and my breasts were gone!

Gone girl!

Twenty days after discovering lumps, and I had tissue expanders sewed into my body.

Does my womanhood reside in my soul, in my brain, in my body, where?

What makes a woman a woman?

Ah, this identity-crisis is multi-faceted, not merely writer-centric, not merely cancer-stricken.

* * *

The surgery went well.

I woke up and saw Tim right away. (My mom and sister were with my kids.) Basically, it was a pretty good experience. We actually laughed a lot. "We'll take the skin off my butt and put them on your boobs, and—in this way—we really will be one flesh," Tim said.

I'd be lying if I said I'm not worried he's going to be sexually repelled by me. He seems immune to such thoughts, though my own dark cynicism keeps me thinking he's faking it for my sake.

Fake on, dude. Fake on.

During the last few days, he's taken me to the bathroom (*I can wipe my own butt, thank you very much!*), regularly drained a disgusting bloody fluid out of bulbs attached to where my breasts once were, propped me up on pillows and slept next to me—waking if I say a word. He's fed the kids, kept them busy, taken care of the cats he hates (their wet food is "worse than cancer"). I can't imagine being without him, and I'm so sad he's had to do this for me.

So here we are.

13

4

Frankenstein Isn't Disney (July 27, 2015)

We are headed to the Happiest Place on Earth (the one in Florida), and I am thinking that I might've—*I just might have*—ripped open one of the scars scritch-scratched across my breasts, scars that are almost like the writing one sees on the inside of block cells, the kind that prisoners make by digging into the cement with the hidden forks they bury inside mattresses. Counting days, keeping track of time. I think I did it, ripped open my own marks. It feels like I did. But it takes too much effort to get up and go check in that pocket-sized airplane toilet. Better to bleed, slowly, probably not to death at this point. There's this sensation of meat ripping.

You've seen it before, carnivores: pieces of steak, stringy, pulling apart.

We are like steak, yes? Or are we like chicken?

What is our texture inside, beneath the skin?

This is the sensation I just felt when I made a small move, just a tiny motion—nothing crazy—on this plane to Disney World, husband and kids in tow. Really, I'm the one in tow. *They're* taking me.

What else could we do?

Who knew mom would get cancer?

I'm dragging my sorry ass to Disney World, and it's quite possible that a scar has ripped open.

It's Stage Two, that's what they told me. Cancer was in one of thirteen lymph nodes. I barely know what that means. What I think it means: *The cancer made it out into the rest of my body. Barely. But it did. It was, initially, just in the breasts—but it found the tunnels and it made it.*

In other words, I'm going to die.

Listen, I've got a plan.

I have to make it till my kids are adults. I can't leave my children mother-less now—not yet.

(My mom told me these statistics she read—she's always reading stats about cancer or mad cow disease or the bird flu—and I don't know her source, but this is what she said: 100% of Stage One people survive, 93 percent of Stage Two people survive . . . and then, then, *I didn't listen since I'm Stage Two*. Of course, they probably only survive for three to six months. But, according to my mom's statistics, *they say* I have a 93 percent chance of survival. I was the one in eight before; I can certainly be the seven in one hundred now—no problem.)

I am intentionally uneducated, not having touched the "cancer library" that accumulates in our dining room. Still, I have put together a plan. Within this first, radical month of frenetic action—consisting of diagnosis, hospital-ization, double mastectomy, tissue expanders, surgical drains—I have written little of my philosophizing, my contemplations on death. In fact, my readers might tactfully ask: *Where have you been?*

Um, planning my funeral?

Plane-bound, probably bleeding, I'll tell you where I've been.

Formulating, mapping out, creating instruction lists.

Tim and I have had morbid conversations.

"I just want to make it till Melody is eighteen," I've told him. Ten more years. Give me ten more years.

But Tim, in response, said something so horrible that you're gonna die, right along with me. I was *floored/mortified/dejected* but also *grateful* in a se-cret, sad way.

(For a while now, I've wanted us to co-author a book on marriage, filled with our strange shit—but it'll never happen. Instead, there is this: *I give you our book on cancer*.)

We were about to engage in our nightly TV habit (yes, nightly), this era marked by *The Sopranos* (and that's another story altogether—how one's own gruesome tale inevitably meshes with other narratives, so my cancer story is somehow or other mafia-related, a mob hit). And we had this tragic-comic conversation.

Tim: "I know you keep saying, *I have to make it ten more years*, and we're all nodding our heads—but that's, like, the worst situation for me."

Jennifer: "What do you mean, that's the worst situation for *you*?"

Tim: "It may be the best for the kids, but it's not the best for me."

Jennifer: "Huh? What are you saying?"

Tim: "If you make it for only ten more years, you'll die when I'm forty-eight. Then, what? Two kids. Forty-eight. It would be better if you died now. Or just make it."

Yes, I flipped out.

Jennifer: "*Die now?* I should die *now?* So you can find someone else?"

Tim: "That's not what I'm saying. I shouldn't have said anything."

Jennifer: "I can't believe you said that."

More flipping out.

Jennifer: "You want me to die *now, not* ten years from now?"

I know I said some weird stuff, too, like he'd never find someone to marry if I died. *In your dreams,* I might've said. *You? A psycho with two kids?*

Which got him depressed.

That I would say that.

That I would believe that.

That I am capable of thinking that.

Well, Tim, do I believe you'll find someone else?

Hey, you probably will.

But, really, I think I'm the one for you, and you're the one for me—and neither of us is a picnic.

And furthermore . . . .

You can be pretty hot and funny, and you're a good dad—so you might get someone, but—wow!—is she in for a surprise, because you are TOUGH to have a relationship with, and I put in my time.

Yes, I did.

I put in my FUCKING time.

Good luck to you, and good luck to her.

And I will haunt you, motherfucker, till the day you die.

Tim: "I don't want for you to die now. Wendy looks just like you, and she acts just like you, so every time she turned around, I'd be seeing you."

True. My eldest daughter is a replica of me as a child. This worries me endlessly because she's sweet and sensitive, and I am not. I don't want her to lose that, like I apparently did.

More freaking out, followed by *The Sopranos* (in which everyone on the show seemed to have cancer), resulting in a new and improved plan. Twenty years. Thirty years? Can I survive for that long? Is that long enough?

Our plane is descending. Survive my kids' childhood.

But I must not grow bitter.

Because I have a bitterness problem.

Like I can get mean.

I have to stick around for my kids—without bitterness.

Can I do it?

5

The Great Gatsby Isn't Disney (August 4, 2015)

It's over.

I did not rip open any scars.

It wasn't easy, or how I dreamed it would be—but Walt Disney was probably an über-genius and going didn't really hurt anything (though maybe that Primeval Swirl did). The distraction was good. And my kids loved it.

I couldn't have done it without Tim. I keep wondering how long any one man can do this, can carry this kind of burden, an entirely unbalanced burden of a relationship. For what am I giving him right now? What's in it for him? Who would have imagined our marriage would turn out like this?

We had fourteen people there at Disney World with four family units. The units broke up into smaller units all the time. *But not us.* I couldn't leave him. We never split up—except for this one moment at the Animal Kingdom, in which he took Wendy on that Everest ride, and I sat, anxiously, drowning in Florida sweat, hoping he'd come back to me—*please come back to me*—even though going off in different directions is something both of us would easily do in previous lives.

We were once so separate.

If this were that marriage book we're apparently not ever going to write, I'd talk about a bizarre phenomenon that's marked our relationship. My guess is that we've spent more time together than almost every other couple I personally know. Much of it has been bad (cancer, for example)—but it's morphed, over the years, into a strange sort of quality-time, in which we've learned each other's moods and habits, adapted, acquired our own language, sharpened an unorthodox and surreptitious humor, and, well, survived. But that's that *other* book. The unwritten one.

Back to cancer, which is probably killing me.

So, first, you might want the Disney-assessment, which is—of course—part of any good cancer story.

What was Disney like? After all, cancer happens to an individual mired in real-time, in a particular historical and cultural context. A little critique?

Peter Pan's Flight and Splash Mountain!

"The Festival of the Lion King"!

I need to confess something from the onset: I still have strong positive feelings about the Muppets.

When you're at Disney World and you're dying, you inevitably find yourself asking an important question: *How do I take this Disney adventure and weave it into my cancer narrative?*

The answer is Michael Jackson. (A note from the future: This was written in August 2015, prior to 2019 revelations about Jackson.)

Allow me to explain.

Epcot was our designated park for my daughter's eighth birthday. We began with this wild princess breakfast, replete with all your favorite princesses. Then, we did it. Did the park.

Look, I'd never seen *Captain Eo*, and I wanted to see it before I died and—for whatever reason—Disney still plays it.

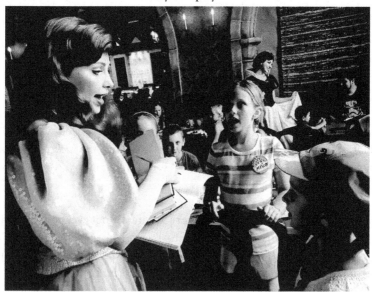

Melody really believes she's meeting a princess. Photo by the author.

Tim said, "You ruined Epcot by making everyone go see *Captain Eo.*"

But that film might be the crux of Epcot: There's something passé about it all, the slight—albeit nostalgic—stench of missing the mark.

Epcot has the stench of missing the mark.

Remember when space was all the rage?

And no one saw the Information Age coming?

"Spaceship Earth"? Really?

I felt all *Mad Men*, all *The Way We Were*.

Of course, I love *Mad Men* and *The Way We Were*.

But still.

The very worst part of Epcot was the very saddest part of Epcot: *Captain Eo.*

By the way, Michael Jackson, supposedly the world's greatest pop star, is dead.

Don't that beat all?

(If there's a pun in there, it's only mildly intended.)

So think like I'm thinking.

Wasn't this a subtle commentary on, another kind of thematic worrying over, the American Dream? And weren't we re-telling *The Great Gatsby* in our Disney playground? Our own true Gatsby, our own beloved Michael Jackson, now dead—like Jay. Our fantasies, embodied in this sweet relic of a film—now defunct.

We forever chase after the green light?

I chased, chased, chased that green light through Disney World—holding onto Tim's hand, breastless, breathless, pursuing my past and my family, racing through the pavilions and showcases of the World.

But *Eo.*

It's all so *Eo.*

The world's greatest pop star was—*if you can believe it, whities*—a black man. A Black Man! But the black man, for some mysterious reason, was turning into a white man. My kids thought *he* was a *she*, anyway—which fits into the whole transgender narrative of today. *So what does this all mean? How problematic is our story?* And why is Disney still showing this outdated film, if not to make us get weepy and sad, especially if one has cancer and is trying to stay alive for a couple more decades? And why not go with something like Pixar and retire *Eo* to its rightful place in cinematic history?

Poor, sweet, fucked-up Michael Jackson!

Dead!

What happened to you, that you should go from the Jackson 5 to this warped *Great Gatsby* figure, this no-man, this every-man, neither black nor white, neither male nor female?

Are we all Gatsbys?

Am I Gatsby?

Maybe this is the lesson we learn at Epcot. We are not poised on the edge of a miraculous future, as Epcot would have you initially believe. Rather, we are reading and re-reading the Great American Novel.

Distraught chasers of the light.

You might be able to see why Tim said I ruined Epcot by making us all go to *Captain Eo*.

* * *

So, yeah, over the course of five days, we went to two—two!—character breakfasts: a Mickey-centric one and the princess one for Melody's birthday. I had so much fun that I almost forgot about my breasts.

There were some special cancer moments.

Like when a couple of the nieces and nephews couldn't help but stare at my chest as they first approached me for a hug. *Hello, Aunt Jennifer!* (I'm a terrible aunt. I always expect people to be excited to see *my* kids, but then I forget to be excited to see *theirs*.) I saw them, my nieces, my nephews, just kids, moving towards me, unable to resist taking a quick glance at my boobs— my Gatsbyfied, green-light boobs. And, for some reason, I felt the shudder of shame, the spectacle of embarrassment.

Like when I forgot to wear my fake breasts when we went to Hollywood Studios one night, and I just wore a tank top and a little bra over my tissue expanders. I whispered to Tim on the shuttle, "I forgot my boobs!" (The next day, when we were about to leave for a park, Tim reached over to touch one and said, "I see you're all set up.")

Like when I had my Merida Moment. I've been suffering quite a bit of anxiety over chemo—more so than I expected. Part of it is this: *What should I do with my bald head?* Strangely, I found myself jealous of Merida in *Brave*. What if I preemptively shaved my head now, in the four days I have prior to chemo, and start wearing a Merida wig? We did, after all, buy Wendy one from Goodwill last Halloween. I bet we still have it somewhere in the garage.

But the Big Cancer Moment: *Insomnia.*

For the first time in my entire life, I had insomnia. I think I slept less than six hours over a five-night period.

I staggered after Tim like a Walker from *The Walking Dead*.

Have you seen *The Machinist*? That was me, too.

"Keep checking on me if we aren't holding hands to make sure I haven't collapsed," I told him.

I was exhausted all day, every day. By 4 p.m. on Friday, I was also paranoid and a little deranged. "I'm going to stroke out on the operating table," I said, speaking of my surgery to put in the chemo port right after we returned to Phoenix. "I'm not gonna make it," I said. "I think I'll die, after all."

I was also afraid to be away from him (it's come to this!).

Every Day: Where The Fuck Is Tim?

(That's a good alternate title for this book: *Every Day: Where The Fuck Is Tim?*)

Another thing about insomnia: You get scared—scared you won't ever sleep again.

I tried to explain it to my brother-in-law and father-in-law like this: Imagine two iPhones glued into your body. Each movement you make, every sleep position you try, is calibrated to minimize your awareness of the iPhones.

But you always fucking know that the iPhones are there.

And that, my friends, was Disney!

Should I die on Monday, at least we went to Disney World.

And I finally saw *Captain Eo.*

6

Unanswered Questions

A Chapter for the Cancer Library (August 9, 2015)

*P*ause. *Deep breath. Where are we?*

I returned from Disney, sleepless, on August 1 (a Saturday).

In the week that would follow, I would go in for outpatient surgery to put in a port (a semi-permanent catheter-thingy installed into a large vein, used for chemo so they don't need to keep poking me: THEY HAD A HARD TIME WAKING ME FROM SURGERY). After the port, I would begin chemo. Then, Tim and I would celebrate our eleventh anniversary on August 7, 2015. Here's the timeline:

August 1, 2015: Return from Disney World, in desperate need of sleep

August 3, 2015: Outpatient surgery for port, drug-induced fabulous sleep

August 4, 2015: Went for preemptive buzz cut and bought a wig, a red one

August 5, 2015: First round of chemo

August 7, 2015: Our anniversary, Mexican food

Here are some concrete facts to include in your own cancer library, now that the week is over.

* * *

Chemo

It's too soon to say what it's like. Mostly, I feel woozy.

Some women don't have chemo. Bitches.

We're watching this documentary streaming on Netflix called *Tig*, about Tig Notaro. She's a comedian who's been through the breast cancer debacle. She's not for everyone (you were warned). But there's something I do find very, very interesting about her: this turning tragedy into humor, and what it all says about Art.

I'd like to do that. Cancer into Art.

Tig.

No chemo.

Me.

Chemo.

Why do I have to have it?

It was, like, a *given*.

Here we go, Jennifer's venture into the scientific . . . .

The lymph system is like the veins and arteries in your body, but it's not carrying blood. Rather, the lymph system carries the garbage filtered out of your blood. Unlike the veins and arteries, there's no heart pumping the stuff out. The lymph system doesn't rely on a pump; it relies on movement and gravity.

The lymph nodes in the armpit are the key in breast cancer, because the garbage/cancer stuff needs to pass through the lymph nodes in the lymph system in the armpit to get to the rest of your body. Tim—I have yet to clarify—is a lung cancer researcher/chemist (hence the goggles and lab coat in the beginning), and he has tried to explain it to me. (If you can believe it, I am married to a scientist who specializes in cancer; he has a degree in chemistry or biochemistry—something like that.) I still don't get it. It sounds like these lymph nodes are countless, infinite. "It's like a meeting place, a pond, in which the rivers stream out from there to the rest of the body," he tried to explain. So, for my cancer to spread, it would need to make it to the pond in the armpit, all ready to move on.

Tim's response to my scientific explanation: "People will forgive you for messing this up."

But how am I messing it up?

The surgeon, during the mastectomy, takes out a little sample of the lymph nodes (this removal of lymph nodes is a big deal, with potential side effects—namely, lymphedema). The doc took thirteen out from me.

Why thirteen?

I don't freakin' know.

It sounds like you get what you get. They just cut out a section, and the pathologist counts the nodes. Most women get something like ten to fifty cut out.

Out of my thirteen, one tested positive for cancer. So, the cancer just made it into the pond.

Bottom line: the cancer was not contained in my breast.

So I'm going to die.

I'm not handling this well, no matter what anyone thinks or the "brave" face I put on. I'm having chemo because—let's be totally honest here—*the cancer made it out.*

Statistically, though, I'm told this is good.

Only one in thirteen! Hooray!

Had the cancer *not* made it to the lymph system, I might've been Stage One. But it did. So I'm Stage Two. Statistically speaking, not much cancer was making it out of the breasts. Just a little.

Well, that answers one question.

* * *

The Wig Decision

I made this decision quickly.

Though I admire—fiercely—those able to go bald, there is a reality to who I am, and who I've always been.

I want to be *Bad Ass.*

I want to be *Rock n' Roll.*

I am neither of these things.

It's cowardice, folks. That's why I'm wearing a wig. Despite my love of nonconformity, I am a conformist. I'm not brave enough to go bald.

I want to walk into my freakin' Starbucks, and I want to be anonymous.

(Do you know that my old Starbucks really did have something to do with this decision? I thought about going in there to write, daily, like I've done this past year—and I realized that I couldn't handle the baldness, the standing out, the possible pity, the concern. I want to blend in at Starbucks.)

Even scarves say, *Cancer!*

I don't want to say it.

So, with little adieu, I cut off all my fake red hair (for which I was "famous") and I bought a wig. That husband of mine just stood right by me!

Kissing his dreams goodbye.

I don't really know what he was thinking.

But my kids.

When I told them that I was contemplating shaving my head—going all Melissa Etheridge, all Sinead O'Connor—I could see the look in their small faces: fear, repulsion. *Terror.*

I couldn't do it to them.

The wig cost $200, and it wasn't covered by my insurance.

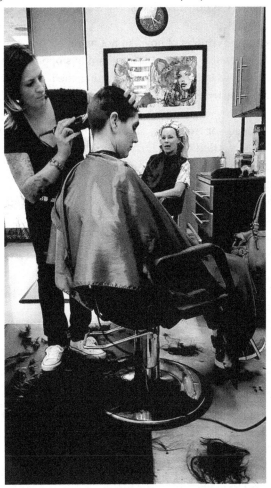

Stylist Krissy Moore has agreed to help me get a part in the *Road Warrior* **re-make. Photo by Tim Bell. Used with permission of Kristina ("Krissy") Moore and her aunt.**

* * *

Bravery

So far, this is the biggest and most widespread farce of them all. I'm only doing what needs to be done. If there's any hint of nobility on my part, it's in my attempt to not get bitter.

And, while we're on the topic, I should say that even my "fight" against cancer is not noble; it is only necessary.

I write. That's it.

Here are some examples of how I'm not noble:

All of the extended members of my family stopped sending us birthday cards and shit when I stopped celebrating their milestones after only three months into marriage. That's right: *I'll forget your kids' birthdays and graduations.*

I demand loads of free time, as well as help with all housework and kid-schlepping—even though my husband makes 90 percent of our income. Because I'm an *Artiste*. Understand this: *I need my creative space.*

My house is only moderately clean, and there are dead cricket parts in my kitchen because I can't pick them up post-chemo, and everyone else mysteriously doesn't see them. The point? *You can't eat off my floor.*

I'm an adequate teacher.

I'm lousy at social plans, at keeping in touch with old friends, and with bringing gifts to people with new babies or new jobs.

I'm bad at bringing friends meals when someone is sick or in the hospital. I've never made a casserole in my life.

I like going on school trips to museums, but I'd rather not make copies or volunteer on field day.

Finally, I'm a so-so mom.

I write.

Brave, I am not.

Do you know the kind of quality people who've swooped in to help me? Quality *women*?

What makes these women so *good*?

So, if through this, I can speak truthfully about the experience, therein rests any smidgen of nobility or bravery.

That's it.

I would like to help other women who are going through cancer, in the way some women have helped me.

I'm sorry I never brought you a meal when you had your baby.

I suck.

* * *

Sex

Yes, we did.

Though we've both had better.

This is where it comes in handy to have been married for a while, because one can just go with the absurdity of the situation and not get too bent out of shape (ha!) on how downright sad the whole thing is. You can just laugh and say, *Not bad for the first time,* or *Well, at least we tried.* We might've given each other a high-five afterwards. But I don't fully remember, because I immediately took nausea meds.

I'll spare you the details, except to say that my heart goes out to the single women in the world or the women going through this alone, not because you're missing all this great sex (because both of us probably would've preferred to watch another episode of *The Sopranos*), but because I imagine that this is so scary, so lonely, so horrible for you. I'm sorry. Other women, other cancer "survivors," can help a lot—but I'm not sure it's what a woman wants.

What does a woman want?

As for sex, I'll also say this. I do feel disconnected from my body. I don't want to see it. I hate looking in the mirror. My kids haven't seen my scarred chest. I sleep with a skullcap on, like I'm all gangster. My body feels like the enemy, and I don't want to have much to do with it.

Gangster.

Going Gangsta.

* * *

My kids.

They're OK.

They don't fully get it, of course—but I think they've felt loved and secure so far. I have—and this is amazing—a plethora of great moms surrounding me. Plus, we moved right before the diagnosis, so Grandma is next door (through the magic bookcase, my own Lenny, a personal Squiggy). I have it good.

(We sold our house and moved into my childhood home right before the diagnosis. This was not easy for me; psychologically, I felt weird about "moving home"—but I was also worried about my elderly mom's future. The time was upon us, or would be soon enough: so we acted preemptively. My mom, a widow since 2002, used whatever money she had to build a guest house in her backyard, complete with a bookcase passageway into our house. *The irony: I got cancer immediately after we moved in, so who was going to help whom?*)

If cancer doesn't kill me, living this close to my mom certainly will.

* * *

Ashkenazi Jew

I had genetic testing done right after the diagnosis.

Because: *I'm a full-blooded Jewish girl, raised by full-blooded Jewish people who converted to Christianity when I was little.*

Your basic Jew for Jesus.

Except my parents fell in with the non-charismatic, no-hand-waving, good-old-fashioned-Protestants-straight-out-of-the-John-Calvin-fan-club crowd.

Let me repeat this, because it's particular and weird—and it's why I'm *almost* really funny but not *that* funny: I'm ethnically Jewish, religiously Christian.

My dual identity has profoundly complicated my life. Sometimes, I try to be all Jewish to get in on the humor—but then I usually end up resorting to my Christianity, which is my more natural self.

(Tim, the biggest goy in the world—with all his pollutant-like mayo—loves to play up how much of a Jewish girl I am.)

The wild thing is that people can sniff me out. The Jews know I'm not the real thing. They can tell I'm faking. The Christians, too. I'm not fully one of them, either. I lack that certain something; I reveal a little ethnic tinge, a bit of a non-WASP edge. I try to get in on the Jewish jokes, but I often get the boot.

I'm this Jewish-Christian entity, ill-informed about most Jewish rituals, savvy about Christian thought, somehow not so untextured as your basic Evangelical. Unruly. A wayward Protestant girl. A little inner-city. A little Jewish ghetto. Kinda *shtetl.*

Ghetto Jew.

Going gangster.

Genetically speaking, though, I'm 100 percent Ashkenazi: from eastern Europe or Russia or one of the Slavic places.

There is a certain Slavic nuance to my unruliness.

I'm a little *Fiddler on the Roof.*

Basically, Ashkenazi Jews are often genetic carriers for the BRCA gene, which results in uterine cancer.

Great.

I probably wouldn't have thought too much about it, but then cancer hit. And part of my persistent Judaism is my ongoing sense of doom. I was immediately tested to see if I were a carrier, and if I were, there would be a 40 percent chance I'd get uterine cancer—so I'd have to get a hysterectomy, which isn't so wonderful, but worse: I'd pass it onto my girls.

I'd give it to my own children.

I lived with that information for a few weeks, while we waited to see if I were a carrier.

I don't know if I can fully explain how devastating all of this was to me. That I might be the carrier of my children's uterine cancer. That I might put them in the position in which they'd need to decide to have hysterectomies early or not have biological children. That I might carry a death sentence for them in my genes.

So, we waited around, breast cancer happening, to see if I were also a genetic carrier for the BRCA gene.

Would I give my girls uterine cancer?

Would I rob them of the experience of having biological children?

How would I tell them?

When would I tell them?

The results came.

And I am not a carrier.

That is one thing I am not.

7

There's Always Frozen Pizza (August 15, 2015)

The lymph node thing is freaking me out. Can't. Stop. Thinking. About. It.

If my mom's survival stats are the same ones I was just looking at, we're talking five years.

Five years!

A friend of a friend got breast cancer. She lived eight years.

And now she's dead.

I'm going to start introducing myself like this: "Hi, I'm Tim's first wife."

Chemo is happening. Basically, if I'm decoding the pattern of my new life, it's this: Get chemo, feel like shit, recover . . . recover . . . feel OK. Repeat.

I do not think there's been any hair loss yet, though I'm wearing a wig that matches the fake red I've been sporting since I was twenty-eight. I still need to shave my legs just like the old days. I suspect that the hair on the top of my head has stopped growing—because usually, at this point, my gray roots are showing. *And they are not.* My hair is still red, albeit buzzed.

So Tim said, "Wouldn't it be funny if you cut off all your hair for nothing, and you could've just stayed a redhead the whole time?"

Yes, *very.*

"I've gotten used to your buzz cut." He said, despite the fact that every time he enters a room in which I'm present and not wearing the wig, the look on his face says, *Oh, yeah. You have cancer.*

Just when he was on the verge of forgetting.

I'm having other effects. My mouth is exceptionally dry, and there is joint pain in my legs. (When I told Tim about my dry mouth, which felt like an admission of guilt, he told me I smelled medicinal for the first few days after chemo. He hadn't told me this earlier because he didn't want to hurt my feelings. That he had been holding on to this information hurt my feelings.)

I tried to do some normal things this week, like go to a beauty makeover class.

You know how I'm always doing stuff like going to beauty makeover classes.

Getting makeovers and shit.

Except this one was for cancer people, and Tim made me go.

Trying to make the cancer babes feel all beautiful!

Come as you are!

(Come doused in mud, soaked in bleach . . . .)

A good friend went with me, and I did come away with some fabulous new makeup (you get free stuff when you're dying), including Estee Lauder's Advanced Night Repair cream, which I suppose I should use, especially if I plan on having an open-casket funeral.

But, please, cremate me.

It's in writing, Tim: *That's what I want. Ashes to ashes, dust to dust.*

My biggest takeaway, however, from the makeover (did I just say *take-away?*) was the knowledge that we're no longer supposed to wear our blush like Duran Duran did in the eighties.

I seriously did not know this.

No one told me.

I've been wearing rouge since 1983 like Nick Rhodes.

The hardest moment of the class was the wig part, in which the cancer people revealed their shaved scalps in order to try on the free wigs. I took mine off in front of my friend. Jenny was the first person besides Tim to see me like this. She handled it well, looking but not looking, crying a little. It was a hard moment for both of us. A kick in the gut. A reality call. My wig is good, frankly, but there's no getting around the truth when it's off.

I have cancer.

That's what my head says.

It was a bit too much for both of us.

I put my wig back on, ready to go. "No. Mine is good." I got all flippant, all nonchalant, feeling the weight of my illness upon our night of post-Duran Duran makeovers. "Girls on Film" had given over to "Women with Cancer."

I did, though, stop wearing my skullcap at night in front of the girls, which I had been doing. Melody didn't blink an eye. Wendy stared a little, but she got over it. Tim always gathers himself together quickly after he first gives me the *oh-yeah-you-have-cancer* look.

But the big cancer highlight of the week has to be the Meal Sign-Up Challenge. I need to give pseudonyms to the people involved, so as not to reveal their true identities. Can we please please please refer to them as *Effervescence* and *Joss*? I've wanted to use those names in my fiction forever, and no one ever lets me. I always get stopped, and someone always says, *You can't do that! How many Effervescences and Josses do you see running around?*

Not many.

Not many at all.

But can we do it here?

I've also been dying (!) for a forum in which I can discuss my teaching experiences of the last few years—and this may be it. Finally!

(Somehow, this might get back to Effervescence and Joss.)

I left college-teaching in 2013 in order to teach seventh grade and high school at a small, very conservative school with a religious affiliation. Though I'm pro-religious affiliation, teaching kids under the auspices of religious affiliation is just not my circus. Or my monkeys. It's just that I'm too shtetl or something.

Did you know that seventh-graders are usually twelve-year-olds? Some have just turned thirteen?

Why didn't I know this?

Why did I think they were little adults interested in great literature?

I should've known, but somehow I didn't.

My own children were still little, and I mostly remembered what being a kid was like by seeing my kids maneuver in their worlds. I did not remember my seventh-grade self.

So I was surprised to find myself, a college teacher, in a room filled with kids who hated reading.

During my brief tenure with these kids (it had the whiff of temporality from the beginning), I came to a bunch of highfalutin conclusions about the differences between college profs and elementary/secondary education teachers. We college profs are "scholars" (use it loosely, my friends, use it *loosely*)—myopic, possibly self-absorbed, in it for the subject matter. In contrast, the teacher types are, well, teaching "experts," classroom managers (I was always, like, *whatever* in my approach to classroom management), kid-friendly, in it for *education*. Which is somehow different from being in it for *the subject matter* (But I should say this: They seem like a generous, philanthropic, happier group than my college colleagues.)

I was not very good at it, to be completely honest.

I don't even like kids, except for my own.

And Tim says that I don't even like them.

(*Not true, girls.*)

I have no managerial skills. Bossing people around is something I can do, however.

Besides floundering miserably at all aspects of my job, I also unhappily gave up the writing as I mentioned earlier (because those teachers honestly do put in the hours and they have no time to write or garden or hike or bake or raise pigeons) and I gave up most of my identity, also mentioned earlier. I missed my myopia, my obsession with fiction. I missed college kids with tats and piercings and dumbass music and weird, angsty views on the world. I missed them fiercely. They were, in part, fodder for my writing.

Which I wasn't doing.

I had run-ins over censorship and James Baldwin and *Lord of the Flies.*

I unhappily took *The Book Thief* off my reading list.

I looked awful, too. Dowdy. There was this other odd phenomenon in which I unwittingly gave up my physical appearance, as well. (Tim didn't notice. "You look the same," he said.)

And this persisted till I was just plain lousy and disliked by a whole slew of seventh graders.

I'm afraid it was mutual.

Well, I rushed back to college after one year.

I spent one year teaching part-time.

I meant to go back to full-time college-teaching this year.

Right on schedule, I got cancer.

What does this have to do with the Meal Sign-Up Challenge?

Well, chemo does slay you, and so I was approached by numerous people to schedule meals, and I shooed them away. *That's why they make Ensure™, guys.* Effervescence and Joss, though, were on me; they wanted to schedule two (!) meals per week from among my friends.

I was, like, *What friends?*

(Tim: "Never refuse free food.")

I tried to stave off Effervescence and Joss. This is deep rooted. I have a super hard time accepting help, which requires humility and grace—things I tend to lack. I hate not doing for myself. I hate needing others so much. I hate my dependence, my neediness.

And I'm sure that this is why my cancer is part of a Grand Scheme.

Is this OK to talk about?

Cancer needs to make sense to me. That seems so horrible to say, doesn't it? Can it ever make sense? Is it just bad luck?

I got cancer for a reason.

(Just so Effervescence and Joss could make me dinner?)

In the Big Picture, I see that it is necessary for me to *humble* myself. I have clung to my identity—you see it here over and over, of course: me pounding you on the head with my damn identity—so fiercely, so unapologetically.

Now, here I am, falling down on aching legs, names of good friends slipping my mind (it happened!), wanting Tim around twenty-four/seven when I've always thought that I'm the one taking care of him.

So a meal sign-up?

Like, *others* will take care of *me*?

And, get this: Effervescence and Joss are moms from the freakin' school that I flunked out of!

Effervescence!

Joss!

Slow down!

I have frozen pizza!

The next thing I knew Joss had a website going—like, she erected a website in an hour—and she was asking every person I knew to bring me food (including people from my past, as well as nice acquaintances) in this warped version of *This Is Your Life*. She wanted to know our allergies, our likes and dislikes. I had to disclose that we sometimes go to Village Inn, and gift cards would be accepted.

Who likes to admit that they like Village Inn?

Effervescence and Joss have been revelatory.

I'm totally flabbergasted—no exaggeration—by the skills involved in such organization. I don't have these skills. It's affected how I am as a wife and mother. And this reveals, mostly to me and now to you, that I couldn't pull it off (this care and nurturing of another), because I have had, quite literally and figuratively, my nose buried in a book.

Effervescence and Joss have revealed my dependency on others. Do I need such intensive help?

Oh no!

I do!

I have cancer!

Effervescence and Joss reveal my lack of vested interest in others: despite my writerly profession, and despite my so-called Artistic Temperament, which is supposed to mean I'm sensitive and shit. My friendships are thin. Not that I'm a bad friend. Rather, I only have a few friends. And my so-called Artistic Temperament (my prized self-identity) has taught me to say, *Who gives a damn if people like me or not?*, rather than learning how to be sensitive to others. My so-called Artistic Temperament has allowed me to isolate myself in the name of Eccentricity. I've gotten away with a lot.

There's Always Frozen Pizza (August 15, 2015)

My eccentricity, my myopia, the feeding of self.

I see the commitment to serve *in others*, the real conviction others have.

And I guess I don't have it.

So, there you go. The meal plan is now in effect.

Basically, I want to apologize to everyone for their kindness, and for my cancer.

* * *

Here's some extra mid-August sex info for you: Did you know that people undergoing chemo are supposed to have protected sex for a few days after treatment, because the chemo can—through bodily fluids—affect a partner?

I know Tim would get so mad if *he* went bald because of me.

Let me go in for another round of poison.

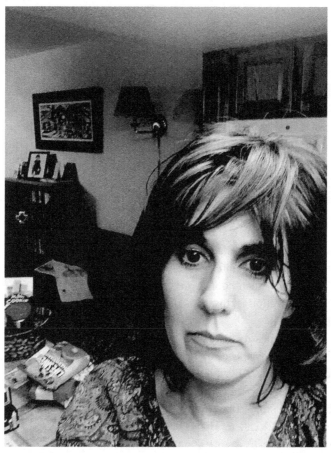

That's the best my hair has ever looked, and it's a wig. Photo by the author.

35

8

Knock, Knock, Who's There? (August 18, 2015)

One can't always be funny.

I'm craving my mask, my fiction, my covering. Something I can hide behind and use to say the sad things. I write sad fiction. Fiction fraught with sorrow. My novel, unpublished as of this writing—will it ever be published now that the author is "having cancer" (as my eldest daughter puts it)?—is dark, unfunny. Not good for the beach.

But my nonfiction is humorous, yes?

I put a spin on darkness—I write of cancer, this unexpected but expected, disaster. My fiction lacks the spin.

Which, then, is the real me?

The funny one in nonfiction, or the dark one of story?

Does Jennifer, not quite riddled with cancer, exist under a cloak?

Is fiction *truer* than nonfiction?

The real question is this, though: *Why are there no gray hairs on the top of my head?*

Yesterday, I heard the story of a "survivor." (I am not yet among the "survivors"—they may need to do a white blood count first.) There are many, many survivor stories. They fill the cancer library. Books and books.

His story was about his hands.

My favorite story about hands is in Sherwood Anderson's 1919 classic, *Winesburg, Ohio*. It's called "Hands."

But this was really a story about fingers.

During chemo, this survivor's fingers curled, and now it hurts him to unfurl his digits. Hands rendered useless. Though he lives—he survived—he now has mitts, paws in digit-shapes. No one would know, because he looks fine.

He has survived.

And I cannot run to him; I cannot hound him with my questions, my inquiries: *You can't type, can you? You don't try to type at all, do you? But you are not a writer, are you? While you were ailing—for we "ail"—what did you do with your time? Did you read weird books, gush aloud on paper, have tragicomic conversations with your husband who is both your life and your death? Is that what you did? Did you pray your sad prayers? Did you try to decipher your beliefs, downtrodden, predestined, hopeful and hopeless? What did you do? How important are your fingers? Are you still alive without your fingers?*

I cannot go to him, this survivor. He is an old man. But his hands, his hands.

Oh God, his hands.

I cannot lose mine.

When you tell me it's temporary, I tell you, *I don't care.*

Maybe my fingers will seize. And this flurry of words will pause. Then, I will truly ail.

Then, I will understand what it means to ail.

Some of my material isn't very funny. There are other things, too—secret things. How to write about the secrets without my cloak of fiction? Those moments when my husband and I sit there, side-by-side, engulfed by our new reality. *We were not ready. We needed more time.*

What is not funny.

I had to ask Tim to stop putting me to bed. It was an elaborate procedure, my bedtime routine. I was propped up on pillows, imprisoned on my back, mostly sleepless. There I was: breastless, pained. Tim checked my angle, my incline. He kissed me goodnight. And he went off to do his late-night ablutions, his email, his worldly matters.

"I have to ask you to stop," I said, one night.

The sorrow of it, the asexuality of it. *He had to stop.*

Should I fictionalize this?

That is not funny.

I think about my experiences: *I know I am built for pain.* I think about this when I am alone. When I'm contemplating life. *I was built for suffering.*

Does this sound arrogant?

You think me vain for saying so?

I know I am able to endure longstanding disappointment.

I can take the unhappiness of not getting what I want.

But can Tim?

This is how I live, the way I muddle through alone, trying to find God in the side effects.

But Tim?

I am built for such a life.

I am built for such sorrow.

What about him?

Should I fictionalize this?

This is not funny either.

Do not imagine what it is like for a bald woman without breasts to approach her husband sexually. Do not picture it. Do not philosophize about inner beauty or strength of character. Do not tell me to think positively. Why do you think I joke?

Think not, also, of the poor husband, robbed of a partnership, teetering from a lack of equilibrium. Now, if glum for one day, the cancer patient *reels*. Just *reels*. Demands that he get a grip, pull himself together, be strong, take care of her—even if she seems OK and was last seen in the kitchen. Always, he must be ready with the charm, the wit. No bad days allowed for him. *Glumness, be gone!*

Tim must be there for me, perpetually happy, persistently optimistic, not tucking me in, not immune to me, not false with me, and not too honest with me, either—because I don't want to know how he's trying, how he's trying so hard, but he can't escape the reality, the truth of my cancer. And what he's really lost is the ability to tell me the truth.

Lest he hurt my feelings.

What he's truly lost is his best friend.

Can he tell me I smelled medicinal for the first few days after chemo?

Can he tell me that my mouth is so dry that a kiss is like sucking cotton?

Can he tell me he just doesn't feel like jumping around and making the kids laugh and telling me it's OK, it's going to be OK?

Can he tell me that he just wants to be alone for a little bit?

Now that my bandages are removed, the scars are no longer Frankensteinian hashtags. They are lines, negative signs. *Canceled out!* That's what I think when I see them.

Canceled!

Subscription over!

Should I fictionalize this?

Not funny.

My insecurities are bottomless, unquenchable.

I follow Tim's gaze to see where it lands.

I watch for eye contact between him and any girl.

I get in there, into his head, and he knows it, and he hates it. This creeping inside his mind to make my judgments. Did I see a spark there with that girl? A moment? An exchange? That pretty girl with her pretty face and cancer-free breasts and hair pulled back: *Did you guys just stare into each other's pupils, unintentionally, maybe—but did it happen?*

And what is *in* that moment?

An acknowledgment?

A *you-are-hot-and-so-am-I-but-this-is-all-we-get, all-we'll-ever-get*?

Is that what I just saw?

And, now, under this rubric of cancer, without my cloak of fiction, I think, *What if that is what I saw?* What can I possibly do? What can I possibly say? Let me lure you back with my word choice, my knack for grammar?

No, I am resigned to my breastlessness, my baldness, my inability to lure. I am resigned to being the girl tucked in at night.

Funny is easy. Serious is not.

Do you wanna hear the one about the girl who got cancer? The one who keeps staring at her fingers?

9

"Body" Is a Four-Letter Word
(August 27, 2015)

I'm struggling here, trying to find my mojo.

Here are two book titles I especially love, titles I've carried with me apart from what might be within their covers: *Written on the Body* by Jeanette Winterson and *Body Betrayer* by Beckian Fritz Goldberg.

These words, in that order!

When I heard them for the first time, separately, they found places in the recesses, the pits, of my word-loving mind. *Those are titles*! Those are accusations, curses, punches in the gut. I loved them. I still do. Intuitively, perpetually, I knew my life, too, was written on my body. I knew my body, too, was a betrayer. I made those titles mean my own things. I might even need to apologize to the authors.

And now I will contribute my own title: *"Body" Is a Four-Letter Word*.

It's not as good, but I like it.

Bodies are physical things. I know something about mine: *My body is failing me.*

The loss of hair under the reign of chemo might be more devastating than having my breasts severed. Would you believe that?

Showers are criminal.

The hair coming out in clumps. I could—if I wanted to—stand there, rubbing my scalp till I was bald. But I stop, at some point. I stop. After the basin is carpeted in hair, the drain clogged in red, I stop. I could go on. I think about it. Just rubbing till it's all gone. But I stop. Why do I? Weariness? Curiosity? Self-loathing? I stop. Tentatively, I get out of the shower, afraid to towel-dry my scalp. I don't want to see the towel. And I'm afraid to look in the mirror. But I do.

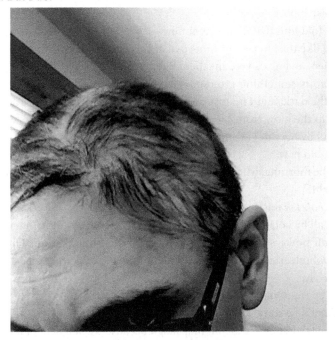

Photo by the author.

Every time, I do.

Each morning, my pillow is like the floor of a hair salon. Tim has had to vacuum the couches. The kids are complaining about hair all over the house. *Look, I wish I didn't have cancer*, I scold Wendy, *but I do. Rinse the shower.*

I had a lot of hair.

Always.

Lots of hair.

I still have some left, but it's only a matter of time now. The red, gone. The red I played up, the colored locks. My falsified hair. My falsified person.

Gone.

Red is not serving me well. I used to say, with comic intention, that I'd stop coloring my wild tresses when Tim went bald. I was waiting for him. Then, only then, I'd give into gray.

But the joke is on me.

Now, with my scraggly remains, the wisps of a buzz cut here and there, would you like to know what I look like, what it is you're not seeing?

Tim hasn't seen it, either; I wear a scarf till bedtime and demand that the lights are off when I unravel myself. In the dark, exposed, I try not to envision how I must appear.

I've told him that it's different now—it's not like it was. I don't want him to see me like this. In a short time, two or three days, I'll be entirely bald, like a little alien, and he can see me then. But not now.

There is something grotesque about it. The patches. I wake with him there in the dark, and I'm unsure if he's looked at me when I was asleep. Has he held up the glow from his phone and examined the creature asleep (momentarily) by his side? He might have.

I would have.

In the morning, when we wake up *very early*, I panic. I shout, "Don't turn on the light!"

I'm not, I'm not, he says.

It'll all be gone soon. And I debate: Do I let it shed till the bitter end, or shave it off now—avoiding the mess, the persistent humiliation? One of my friends, volunteering to help me, said that I might *take charge* and get rid of it preemptively.

I keep thinking of those words, you know? *Take charge.*

Like it'll be some kind of empowerment thing.

If we try joking—and you may laugh because we laughed—I look, right now, in the brutality of this shedding season, like a baby orangutan. Not just a baby orangutan. But a baby orangutan in the Holocaust.

Yes, I look like a baby orangutan in the Holocaust.

That's what is happening.

I could tell you about my decision to have radiation. I planned on writing about that. Or my thoughts on forming an agenda, a mission. I need to add something to this narrative, some kind of missionional thrust. Choose a cause. Like Jimmy Carter. I thought about telling you about teaching college this week, how I went all Betty Draper on the stairs.

That is coming, too. I could tell you about my corpselike color.

Or this: *I got my period!*

Chemo is supposed to push me into menopause. And there it was, right on schedule. When I was on the verge of giving away my stash of tampons! My body is falling apart, doing the whole *Body Betrayer* thing, but I'm still menstruating!

For another day.

Today, close your eyes. Picture this: red hair all over the place, except for on the top of my head.

10

The Shock of Me (August 31, 2015)

Every day, I pray that I live until my children are adults.

Melody has asked, "Are you positive that you'll be better in five months?" (I'll be done with chemo then, so five months has become our arbitrary get-well point—but then it's onto six weeks of radiation. This is another story entirely, because I'm opting for it. It's an *option*.)

The best I can do is tell Melody, "I hope so. I hope I'm better."

And so my children live with a confidence that I will make it. What do you think of this? Am I lying to them?

There. We got the morbid stuff out of the way.

Well, in regards to my no-doubt highly accurate description of myself as a baby orangutan, I need to tell you that the hair-shedding has slowed down remarkably, leaving me—right now—in *Baby Orangutan State*.

I've heard a few things about this. First, just wait till the next chemo treatment. And then it'll go again. Second, sometimes it doesn't all fall out ever. And you're left in Baby Orangutan State.

For some reason—which you might philosophize about—I'm resisting shaving it all off. I'm clinging to what's left, even though I hate it so very much.

Go figure.

I think my friend Lara (of Snotty Literati fame) put it best: "Fully shaving it might make you feel, for a moment, that you're in control . . . of a completely out-of-control situation."

Yes, that's about right.

Not that the smidgen of temporary control wouldn't be a good thing . . . .

There's another part of me that kinda wants to see what happens.

This Baby Orangutan State made me reconsider, however, the part about not showing the family my crazy-ass cancer look.

I will tell you this: *I'm really, really hot.* As in *sweaty hot*—not *sexy hot*.

Which may be an effect of chemo. Or living in the desert. My wig has frizzled a little. Collapse is likely.

Truly, it's a good thing I'm one of the young and healthy ones dying from cancer; my toleration for this wasteland is good.

So I showed the family my head.

What choice did I have?

First, when Tim wasn't home, I tried it out on the girls. Melody didn't give a shit. Wendy was very disturbed initially, trying—obviously—to control her facial expression. I quickly put my skullcap back on. Poor kid!

Later that same day, I took it off in front of everyone.

The shock of me!

Tim responded well. (I still do not know what he's thinking.) This time, though, the girls adjusted, uncomfortably, and asked questions after about an hour (it took them about an hour of side-glances). They wanted to know stuff: *Why is it falling out? Will it grow back? Does it hurt? When will you stop wearing the wig? Will you stop wearing it when your hair is like Mary Margaret's* (Once Upon A Time)?

Guys, I'm never going to look like Mary Margaret.

Tim got slightly impatient with their questions. "How many times are we going to go over this?" he asked.

But I knew: The reality of cancer hit home with the grotesque. And it is grotesque. Let's not pretend otherwise.

They were sad, but Wendy said, "You're lucky because you get to suck on that candy." (Dry mouth from chemo = stash of mints and hard candy.)

And this made me think of Carol on *The Walking Dead*. I love Carol. You love Carol. *Who doesn't love Carol?* She's a nut job, but, c'mon, she's been through a lot. *Can you blame her?*

But that's beside the point.

Her hair.

Even before this cancer debacle, I was a little fascinated by her hair. Short, gray.

Guys, not Mary Margaret but Carol. I will look like Carol.

I'm serious about my fascination with her hair. At first, it was this logistical preoccupation: *How does she keep it so short during the Zombie Apocalypse? Who cuts it for her?* Others were concerned about how the survivors got toilet paper and water, but I wanted to know about haircuts. And then, as my complicated relationship with Carol developed, my own questioning morphed: *And why does she want to keep it so short? Why? Why? Why?*

But deep in my heart, I sensed *alliance.*

Carol and I are sisters.

We are the same.

Go with me into the show. We're in that prison. Was this the third season? The prisoners are dead, except for two hardened criminals. One of them—who will be dead soon—is creeping around Beth too much, and Carol tells him to get away. The prisoner, who's rather gross, says something disgusting like how there are not a lot of female options around—there's Beth and a couple others. Then, he dismisses Carol, saying something about how she's a lesbian, so she doesn't really count.

And Carol says, "I'm not a lesbian."

The prisoner guy says something like, "But your short hair?"

And there I was, thinking thinking *thinking.*

But your short hair?

But your short hair?

But your short hair?

The whole scene, by the way, is done very tactfully. My point: Dumbasses who didn't know her thought she was a lesbian.

Well, moving along—*forget Mary Margaret and Carol*—there is the possibility that my bouts of clammy, fevered, *I'm-so-hot-but-not-like-Mary-Margaret-is-hot* assertions are actually menopausal. Even though I did just get my period. Which was normal but brief, if you must know.

(And here's a note from the future. Written in December 2016: *It would be my last period ever.*)

So Tim said, "Enjoy it while it lasts."

11

Niche, Which Sounds a Little Like Nietzsche (August 31, 2015)

I want to add something to my narrative, so it's not just a book about cancer. (Have you seen all the books about cancer? I need a niche! *Which sounds a little like Nietzsche.*) Get a cause. Be an advocate. There is the do-gooder aspect of this: Work for good, see change. And there is the myopic part: Make a legacy, have a meaningful life.

What might be my philanthropic thrust, besides the obvious: my kids?

Here are some possibilities under consideration:

My own brand of Arts advocacy, which is to say "literature advocacy"?

This is most likely and most personal. First and foremost, we're talking to my own girls: *Be readers, talk about books, experience the Arts, interpret stuff, think about things, do not be afraid of controversy, stop the naïveté.* Second, this is part of my writing vocation, which I hope to do till my demise: *Write fiction and nonfiction up to MY standards.* Third, *I'm pretty concerned about the state of art consumption and production among religious types.* (That old drumbeat: *More Johnny Cash, Less Thomas Kincade!*) Get you all on the U2 bandwagon! Read Marilynne Robinson now!

Education reform?

(It's not gonna happen. Don't worry. Besides the fact that I lack the knowledge, I probably lack the passion. And I'm really only concerned about literature.)

U.S. presidential politics?

Doubt it. Some people totally know this about me, and others don't. I began adulthood in politics, which is to merely say I have a BA and an MA in it, and I spent some time in very low-level jobs in political science-y places with the intention of working in international relations (human rights, civil rights)—though I quickly learned it wasn't going to work since I was short of any real volition, ambition, and interest, *and I wanted to be a fiction writer.* I'm not liking Trump, though. (By the time that this is published, my like or dislike will be irrelevant.) I guess, in truth, I might be more aligned with that eloquent freak, Russell Brand, than I'd care to admit. I just read *Revolution,* his utopian book—with which I don't fully agree. He has some good points, though. *Brand, I just plugged your book—which needs a good edit. I also just called you a freak. All things considered, that's not so bad. I could've done worse. I have done worse.*

Human Rights/Civil Rights?

I'm inclined to keep active on this front in some way, but I need to think about efficacy, and—admittedly—it's secondary to my literary interests—though it's not divorced from my literary interests. You know, it always has seemed to me (and I don't think I'm wrong here), that artists were among the first and the strongest civil rights advocates. (There are probably exceptions?)

Animal rights?

Sorry, guys. Nope. I do think everyone should get a pet. I also think people who kill animals for fun may be psycho. And SeaWorld needs to shut down.

Cancer stuff?

I don't wanna. But I will. For the women. I don't want to get into the kale or the cures so much. I do want to be there for other women, and one of the scary things I've learned through this is that *it's going to happen to some of you.*

I'm sorry, I'm so sorry.

Cancer comes to you. It comes without ceremony.

(Do you know anything about Steve Jobs? I'm not doing heavy-duty research here, but . . . . Following diagnosis with pancreatic cancer, he opted out of immediate surgery and Western medicine. He didn't want his body "opened"—sounds like a man to me—so, for nine months, he did diets, juices, meditation, et al. Then, well, he obviously needed surgery. But it was too late. One of the major tragedies here is that early surgery could've saved his life.)

So, women, this is my very first piece of real advice to you: *If you get diagnosed, get the motherfucking cancer out of you as soon as possible.*

I better stick to books.

Literature.

My agenda.

It's chemo on Wednesday, so I'm in prep-mode, because—in truth— I'm *Mom*, and I'd better prepare. For me, get bananas, Gatorade, Ensure. Buy enough canned cat food. Fill the car with gas. Figure out carpooling for the girls. Do laundry. Check to see if there are bills or correspondence or editing or teaching prep that I can do *now*. Everything must be done *now*.

If I were to die, I have no clue how Tim would keep track of the girls' homework or manage to get them anywhere.

12

I'm Like This Because I'm Doing This (September 6, 2015)

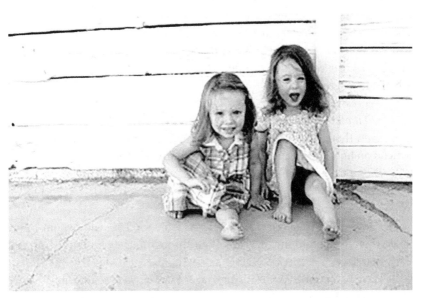

Photo by Lex Treat, photographer. Used with permission.

The routine—for there already is one—is to see my oncologist and get chemo on Wednesdays when I'm done teaching English 101, a dazzling red faux-mop on top of my head. Seeing the oncologist takes ten minutes; chemo, about two hours. Tim and I usually grab lunch beforehand. Subway, our hangout. We are all about the chipotle.

He stays with me during chemo, and we joke around mostly. We are different from how we were in those early years of marriage, now able to balance each other out, all yin and yang, reserving our secret marital weapons (ill-tempered dictatorial tendencies) for another time. In this, we are united: *the illustrious oneness of a cancer-tainted marriage.*

We sit in a room of recliners; they are not uncomfortable, though who wants to sit on anything in a room full of dying people? Some will die sooner rather than later. The recliners are easy to clean, wipeable, great for leaking body fluids, blobs of phlegm. There are, I think, pillows and blankets available—but, unlike other patients, I'm hot all the time. It's the damn rat, this wig. *Why, oh why, can't I be rock 'n' roll? Why the rug?* There are snacks (Keebler?), coffee (*not so good*), and water. TV in some sections. It seems like *Ellen* is always on. We bring our books.

The oncology nurse—a wildly compassionate oncology nurse!—comes over, cleans my port (the surgically installed little knob into my body), freezes my skin, and sticks in the IV needle that is attached to a bag of drugs hanging nearby. I don't feel the needle. First, I get nausea meds. Then, the cancer drugs. I don't know the regimen. Tim does. I asked last time if my chemo is considered *strong, medium,* or *what.* The nurse said, "I'd say *strong.*" Which is what I wanted to hear.

Aggressive.

Kill it all.

Even though my mom just sent me one of her famous Internet cancer articles on how chemo and radiation cause future cancer.

Damn the Internet!

Damn Al Gore!

What choice do I have?

I am buying time. Time for my kids. Time for Tim, with whom I now share this unexpected life, having gotten through our own perfect storm of early marriage.

Have I mentioned our early marriage? How we were so unhappy that we thought we might die?

But we survived; we found each other. And here we are now, in recliners. Kicking back. Tim with Sudoku. Me, novel-enmeshed. *Sounder.* I never read it. I picked up a book on a dog that's going to die.

Here we are, then, in the chemo room, having emerged from a tempest to this cancer business, this calm.

That is not a reference to Shakespeare.

I'm Like This Because I'm Doing This (September 6, 2015)

* * *

Wendy was born on February 21, 2006, to Tim and me—slightly premature at thirty-six weeks. We had gone to a huge used book sale at the state fairgrounds that day. I had a horrible cough. He was sick, too, but we had sex that night anyway at, like, 3 a.m.? (*Really?*) On the toilet, after the requisite pee, I felt something—something that must be labor. Pain. *Really. Bad. Pain.*

We exchanged famous last words.

From my place on the toilet, post-coital, I was doubled-over (as much as I could be doubled-over) and naked. *Don't picture it.* Belly, big. *Not pretty.* I called to Tim in the bedroom, "Tim, could you come here?"

Tim, naked, too (did we really sleep naked once?), responded, "Can *you* come *here*?"

No, I certainly cannot.

"Baby. It's the baby." *I'm having the baby.*

I showered before we left—not wanting to smell like freakin' sex—which must've been painful, and then we left for the hospital. We were ill-prepared, but we wanted her. We wanted a baby badly, so badly—and I wanted a girl.

What did I know about boys?

Who would keep me company in my discontent?

A girl.

I would take her to museums. We would see movies together. There would be trips to the zoo.

I would not be lonely.

Our marriage was really bad.

Tim rushed us to the hospital, and I vomited on the floor of the car in the hospital parking lot. Wendy was born in the wee hours of the morning. I don't remember this, but "Where the Streets Have No Name" by U2 was playing in the delivery room when I had my emergency C-section. It was all very symbolic because of my longstanding relationship with U2. Symbolic, blessed.

And I know all moms think this—but my baby was beautiful.

She was beautiful.

Child of my sorrow, child of my heart.

Wendy Ireland was beautiful.

* * *

Top Ten Wendy Ireland Quotes:

1. When our indoor cat, Jules, ran into the garage, I chased him back into the house. Wendy, alarmed, asked, "What happened? Does he need his shoes?"

51

2. After a bath, Wendy was stark naked and doing ballet stretches in our room. Tim came in to get her dressed, and she said to him, "I'm like this because I'm doing this!"

3. Wendy was watching an old episode of *The Muppet Show*. Miss Piggy didn't appear right away. Wendy wondered where she was. Finally, Miss Piggy showed up, and Wendy declared, "There's that pretty girl."

4. Tim was having a serious conversation with Wendy, telling her that if she felt sad about something she could tell us. Even if we couldn't find an immediate solution, he told her, we'd think about it. "But you can always come to us." Wendy took a moment, thought hard. Dogs were barking outside. She looked at Tim and said, "Can you get rid of those dogs?"

5. She declared, "I don't want to marry a cowboy. Their fiddles are too loud and they dance all around."

6. Wendy announced, "I think leaves are fantastic!"

7. According to Wendy, Eve was created from Adam's "Bungee Cord."

8. I told her that Martin Luther King Jr. wanted us to know that we're all God's children. Wendy added, "And we all use the same bathroom."

9. When Melody asked Wendy to do a puzzle with her, Wendy answered, "I would love to, but I don't want to."

10. She was sitting on the potty, very into her book. I was in and out, asking questions. "Are you done yet?"

    Wendy wanted to continue reading. Finally, I said, "It smells like you're done."

    Shaking her head fiercely, she said, "No, that's just a dead animal."

13

The Cadence (September 6, 2015)

For our wedding, Tim wrote me a poem. "Our Flesh and Cadence."

It was the last poem he would ever write for me.

We turned from cadence to flesh, which sounds sultry and sexy but actually means this: *Every time one of us turned around, the other one was standing right there. Who could breathe?*

> She was beautiful in that setting sun
> and now she's with me, woven
> in wonders beyond our doing
> We drink from the cup that came unannounced,
> hold tightly and rightly to a flame of yearning,
> excellencies hot with motions of youth
> We shall venture in vows, sacred grip
> unleash the flood of love's battalion
> We see the cup that is filled with awe,
> fully contains our flesh and cadence
> and savor the sip that first is given.

* * *

We had a second baby. Another girl! Which is what I wanted *again*!

Melody arrived on July 31, 2007—the night before the planned C-section. My plans have *never* worked. Our marriage still sucked, and our children were shields, warding off the havoc we knew would come one bright apocalyptic day.

We loved them; we loved them dearly.

How did one such as I give birth to two such as these?
Such beautiful girls. So healthy. So perfect.
Our flesh, our cadence.

* * *

I gradually started reading books again after Melody was born. The first book I remember reading was Stephen Colbert's *I Am America*.
It was so good!
Life was a mess. What do people say? *A hot mess.*
What fresh hell is this? I like that one.
Melody's first dolls were named *Baby Lye-Lye* and *Chin-chin*. No clue where those came from. Her all-time favorite stuffed animal was Pink Bunny, who was a bunny who could've passed for an aardvark.
Pink Bunny is a girl.
I still think Pink Bunny is a boy.
I shopped at Walmart. I hated Walmart. Guys approached me in the parking lot. I'd be leaning into the back seat, buckling Melody into her car seat. Wendy would be kicking back in her seat. I'd stand up straight, looking all haggard housewife-ish. There, some guy would be standing. "I'm sorry to bother you," he'd say. "I ran out of gas. I'm wondering if you could just give me a little money to fill up the tank."
"No, I cannot," I'd say. "I'm sorry."
I'd be this admixture of anomalies, a body snatcher, a pretender. Married, but not supposed to be married to this guy. A mom, but lousy at it. Shopping at Walmart, complaining about the smells, dissing the homeless guy, charging up my credit cards, listening exclusively to Prager and Medved—because someone told me that NPR was the voice of the liberals, the communists, and the Devil. I'd be planning on homeschooling, despite my dislike of home or schooling. I'd take my New York/Greenwich Village/liberal think-tank NGO/left-voting/bloated ego/varicose-veined self and tell that homeless guy to fuck off. I'm a stay-at-home mom now, miserably married, child ensconced, and I'm not giving a cent to anyone off the streets. *Get a job, fuck-face.*

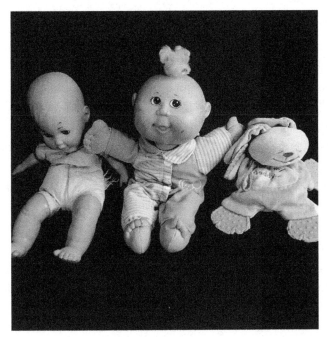

Photo by the author.

* * *

We went to a few different marriage counselors. One strategy they all taught us was to "reflect back" what our spouse was saying to us. So, if Tim said something nasty to me like, "You're a bitch from hell," I might say, "What I'm hearing is that you think I'm a female dog from Hades. Do I have this correct?"

If I were to call him a "motherfucker," he might say, "What I'm hearing is that you believe I am the mom of someone who fucks, or perhaps I am someone who will fuck a mom? Is this correct?"

We had workbooks.

We had "staff meetings."

We read *The Five Love Languages: The Secret to Love That Lasts*. If I remember correctly, Tim's love language was the one in which you were supposed to have sex with him every waking moment, and my love language was the one where you're supposed to tell me how wonderful I am as often as possible.

Tim was always the first to refuse to go for further counseling. He didn't want to pay the co-pay.

* * *

Top Ten Melody Prose Quotes:

1. We were watching one of those nature shows, and a lion was eating some unidentifiable animal. Melody declared, "I think it's a unicorn."

2. I asked Melody to remain sitting on the toilet until I left the room. Melody responded, "No one wants to see poop except for Satan and Wendy."

3. There happened to be a raccoon in our neighborhood. Melody got nervous. "Is the haccoon in the grass? I don't want the haccoon to eat Ju-ju" (Jules, the cat).

4. She would gear up to flush the toilet like it was the wheel on *The Price is Right*. She'd say, "Yo, yo, YO!" Or, "Ach, ach, ACHOO!"

5. Referring to *Beauty and the Beast* as "Beauty and the Beef," Melody asked, "Does the Beef bite?"

6. She was trying to recall Mount Rushmore, so she asked me, "Who are those boys who rule?" I had no idea what she was talking about, so she added, "You know, Barack Obama?"

7. Bosco, the other cat, got very sick. Melody said, "If he dies on my lap, we'll have to change my pants."

8. Tim asked Wendy how many people carried the tabernacle in the Old Testament. Wendy said, "Four!" Melody responded, "You're on fire tonight!"

9. When there was a dead bird on our carport, we heard a bird chirp. Melody quickly declared, "It's the dead bird."

10. She said something about a butt crack. "That's inappropriate language," I told her. Melody responded, "I'm speaking French." Wendy interjected, "That's not French." And Melody answered, "Yes, it is. I know. I'm a scientist."

14

Monsters (September 6, 2015)

Is it enough to say—will it suffice to say?—that we lived through it and came out on the other end? There are the unspeakable parts, and there is recovery.

And that is it about my marriage: *My cancer is invasive; my attitude is evasive.*

* * *

When Melody was fussy, I said, "Melly, why are you crying so much?"

Wendy looked at me and responded, "Monsters."

Tell me about it.

* * *

Somehow, from my place in that fresh hell, I sold a couple books to publishers.

I did a book-signing at a North Phoenix Costco (Costco!), which would likely be my one and only Costco appearance. I sold six copies of *The Freak Chronicles.*

One guy looked at my books, much to the annoyance of his wife. I knew he wasn't going to buy. "So what's the end result of your book?" he asked, which isn't really a bad question.

I paused long enough to dramatically deliver my answer: "Enlightenment. Fulfillment."

Another guy looked at the title and curtly said, "No, thank you."

* * *

Melody asked me to draw her a dinosaur.

I did, and both girls examined it. It wasn't very good.
Wendy declared, "But you sure can draw a horse!"
Tell me about it again.

* * *

What having two books published meant.

It meant you might be able to get away with wearing blue jeans when your workplace called for "business casual." This was not guaranteed, however.

It meant that people who had no clue who you were might be slightly impressed by your accomplishments for approximately three minutes before forgetting you completely.

It meant that people who considered themselves your intimates or even just your acquaintances would have a measure of anxiety when you were around because of one of the following reasons:

1. They hadn't read your books, nor did they want to, and they were afraid you were going to ask.

2. They owned your books but they hadn't read them, and they were afraid you were going to ask.

3. They read your books and they didn't like them, and they were afraid you were going to ask.

4. You're a general pain-in-the-ass who walks around all self-important now, and they were afraid you were going to talk. *About your stupid books.*

* * *

We were parents with young children, and they were sweet girls, so sweet. They didn't toss around creepy kindergarten threats like, "I'm not going to be your best friend anymore." They didn't try to get other kids in trouble.

But they were exposed to cruelty from others.

I saw something once while driving in my car. Wendy and her little friend were in the back seat, and I watched them through the rearview mirror. Wendy had made a picture for this friend of hers—it involved scrap paper and staples. Still, my daughter drew it with fervor and—let me tell you this—*love*. She loved her little friend. More than she probably should have. She possessed the star-struck affections that are, usually, unwarranted and one-sided.

I didn't want her to love too much.

I didn't want her to love too much, lest her love go unreturned.

That would be a particular kind of hurt, the soul-shaping kind.

So, my daughter made this picture. Wendy gave it to her little friend.

They were at that age in which they converse. Five, six? These little kids talk to one another. Mostly, they say silly stuff—nothing profound. But I heard the other little girl tell Wendy that the picture was "kinda garbagy."

Kinda garbagy.

I heard it.

I didn't interject.

Instead, I just watched Wendy's face through the mirror.

Wendy had heard it, too.

The silly conversation with its nonsense and noise had continued, but I could see my daughter's expression.

Her frozen smile.

Her arrested animation.

Her mind working over the hurt.

I could see it and I wanted to go to her, to hold her, to tell her: *It's her, not you.*

But I didn't. I let her experience that anguish, that realization. Should I have intervened?

Another time, Tim took the girls to McDonald's and they were playing on the PlayPlace stuff—despite all my warnings about urine and potential syringes full of heroin. Melody, five, was standing on something. Some kid didn't want her there—so the kid kept pinching Melody's toes (Melody was wearing sandals).

Melody kept getting pinched.

Tim watched.

He watched this kid pinching Melody.

Melody tried to shake the kid off—but the pinching continued.

The thought passed through Tim's head: *Just kick that kid in the fucking face.*

Eventually, Tim moved them along, breaking it up peacefully, no foul language involved. But you have to wonder: *Why the pinching? And what is my daughter to do? Endure the meanness? Turn the other cheek? Not let anyone walk all over her? Ever?*

What damages do we sustain?

When do we fight back?

* * *

I went to a writing conference in Boston.

On my plane, I told a very nice fundraiser sitting next to me that I was a writer. She told me, in turn, "I once high-fived Bruce Springsteen, missed his hand, and touched his chest!"

* * *

I formulated my own rules for writing.

1. Don't write about your husband's family, especially his mother.

2. Don't write about anything you feel it necessary to qualify with the following: "But it really happened."

3. Don't write about masturbation. Because I don't want to hear it.

4. Don't write about the dream you had last night. Because it doesn't mean shit.

5. Don't write about how great your pets are, unless you're talking about my pets.

* * *

How we saved our marriage: We watched *The Office*.

By the summer of 2012, we needed relief. And we discovered that *The Office* was about love.

Dwight and Angela get married while standing in their own graves.

And Jim and Pam!

O Jim and Pam!

Tim said, "If we had the cameras on us all the time like Jim and Pam, we'd have the same great big love story."

* * *

We joke during chemo. It's our way.

We put on a show for spectators.

If people were listening—*they're not*—they'd think we were the funniest people in the place. We're bringing down the house, knocking those chemo patients to the floor. *Man, are we hilarious!*

Sometimes we argue about who's funny and who isn't.

"I'm funny," I'll say. "I'm very funny. Everyone thinks I'm funny."

"No, they don't," he tells me.

"Yes, they do. I'm hysterical. What are you talking about?"

"Only on paper," he says.

"Well," I continue. "It works. I don't talk to anyone. I only talk to you in person. And I'm very funny with you."

"You are not."

"Yes, I am."

Tim *is* pretty funny. People only know this when they're with him one-on-one, though. He's not funny in crowds. *He is so unfunny in crowds that it isn't even funny.* And he wasn't funny during our bad marriage days.

He tells me now, "I don't know how you could stand me."

"I saw the gem buried in the sand," I say. I think I'm trying to tell him that I knew he was a diamond in the rough. Whatever. I'd write it properly if I had a pen.

The chemo nurses laugh with us, because our attitude is so good, and I look great, and Tim looks like some kind of athlete altogether—we're so shiny and healthy and boisterous. You'd never really know that I was dying of cancer and Tim used to be so un-funny.

You'd never know.

Tim reads a book on Arizona history published in 1965. He interrupts my novel-reading and says, "Flagstaff was the EPICENTER of sheep!"

He's all excited and he adds, "Now, it's all coming together."

Followed by, "Oh my goodness!" and "Dude!"

Dude!

But after it's all over and we head out into the sun, he's a little somber. On our way home, I say, "I know it's a lot for you. Watching me have cancer."

15

Who's Got This? (September 21, 2015)

And now I'm thinking of the fragility of it all, the precipice over which we hover, the delusion of control in which we rest.

I just finished grading English 101 essays, a slew of them. This chemo treatment hit me harder than the others, and I couldn't do much besides grade. I could sit on the couch and grade poorly constructed essays about cleaning up house parties, along with a few startling pearls from greenish freshmen. I graded and graded. Melody wanted to play in the living room, and I told her I was in there. She protested: "You've been in there *all day.*"

Grading papers. Being sick.

This was the first time I didn't want to eat anything. I had heard stories—horror stories—about feeding tubes.

But that wouldn't happen to me. I ate! And, then, suddenly, I didn't.

So here I am now: hating every time someone mentions food. *And you guys fucking mention it all the time.* Even hummus, my standard cancer craving, sounds like perversion. I can't make it through a can of Coke.

I sat for days, grading papers. The girls have accepted that daddy is everything now, and mommy sits, bald, in the other room. Tim, ever kind. I still find his deepest thoughts, his fears, a mystery.

I know mine go something like this: *Will I always be like this?*

Sometimes, I try to make him talk. What do I want to hear?

I'm sick of you?

No, not that.

What then?

I'll keep doing this forever?

Is that what I want him to say to me? Some reassurance that he'll just sit by till I die?

At night, on Ambien now, I wedge a pillow along my body in an effort to forget my flesh, my now cumbersome falsies, breasts hard and untouchable. Jokes for boobs. I fall asleep instantly, but then spend the bulk of the night sleeping-waking-sleeping.

I look for Tim in bed—not reaching out to touch him. Oh, no, not that: *Why try? Why suggest such neediness, such dependence, such sorrow?*

One night, I had a nightmare that he asked me, *cordially*, for a divorce. The cordiality was most striking. In my dream, I was all cancered out, going through chemo, and he saw his opportunity for freedom in a few months: He'd wait it out. Like a proper motherfucker. His freedom existed *over there*, in that *other place*. And, in my dream, what could I do? What could I say? I could only *cordially* grant him a divorce.

I had no control.

It was only a dream, but I woke up mad. *Do not leave me*, I would plead. And then I graded more papers.

The kid who told me that things don't happen for a reason and you control your own destiny got a D on his paper. *Well, kid*, I wanted to write on his final grades, *What happened there? Why'd you get a freakin' D?*

Now, teetering on that precipice of self-sovereignty, I'm really struggling with the issue of control. *Who's got this?* Even more critical, I guess, than *why*.

There's "Invictus" by William Ernest Henley:

> Out of the night that covers me,
>   Black as the pit from pole to pole,
> I thank whatever gods may be
>   For my unconquerable soul.
>
> In the fell clutch of circumstance
>   I have not winced nor cried aloud.
> Under the bludgeonings of chance
>   My head is bloody, but unbowed.
>
> Beyond this place of wrath and tears
>   Looms but the Horror of the shade,
> And yet the menace of the years
>   Finds and shall find me unafraid.
>
> It matters not how strait the gate,
>   How charged with punishments the scroll,
> I am the master of my fate,

I am the captain of my soul.

Or is the whole world in His hands?

But what crazy tension exists in this life! If I say that I do not control my destiny, am I advocating passivity? Are we mere victims? Do I roll over and die?

Or am I the captain of my soul? What about these people who keep pushing the "Power of Positive Thinking"? (People keep telling me to think *positively*; even more than the advocation of kale, I am entreated to think *positively*.)

Will my cynicism kill me? Did my stress—I *am* pretty high-stressed— originally feed a cancer cell, giving it life, letting it bloom?

I can see this, you know: Cancer taking root in my breast, growing, growing, *growing*.

I brought it on myself.

Is *positive thinking* the same thing as *hope*?

Is this a theological battle between *free will* and *predestination*? Is there some kind of equation in which one gets four parts of autonomy to every six parts of dependence?

* * *

This recently happened.

All on the same damn day. *Go figure!*

Tim was in a bad mood, a little mopey.

Then, my father-in-law—who has pretty much been the healthy one (ironically, I've kinda been the healthy one, too) until he unexpectedly suffered a stroke about a year ago (he fully recovered)—passed out! A couple of times!

Followed by some seizures! His heart stopped during one of them!

But there was more.

Tim's been wondering if I'd divulge this part, and I told him I would.

Of course I would!

Get ready.

My body is now game, ready for exploitation, a palate on which to paint this cancer picture.

In short, *I saw blood.*

Where?

Yes, there!

On the toilet paper, post-stool.

I didn't tell anyone.

Then, I figured that I should probably tell someone, right?

Tim—the resident poop expert—got right on it.

I called my oncologist, who is required to account for every ache and pain.

My oncologist said, "We need to get blood work done immediately in case your platelets are low. If they are, you'll need a blood transfusion."

And that was when Joe, my father-in-law, had a couple seizures.

Tim *cannot* have a bad day. This was against our cancer rules. He needs to be cheerful at all times.

He had to pretty much pull himself together and take care of his wife who was bleeding out of her ass, while his father was hospitalized because his heart stopped. Tim and I went to the nearest lab to have my blood drawn, while—simultaneously—Joe had a pacemaker installed.

How crazy is that?

Am I the captain, or is the whole world in His hands? Is it some kind of spectrum of sovereignty?

Well, Joe survived—and we're all very thankful and aware of our fragility. The circumstances seemed finely orchestrated. He had been driving moments before, but he passed out at home. He had the seizures in the presence of medical people. *He could've died, but he didn't.*

Back to my bleeding butt!

The platelets were normal, so new equally fun options presented themselves: hemorrhoids or something monstrously called an "anal fissure." I still don't really know what that is, but it sounds like an alien slug that plants itself in your anus and rips you a new one.

I remain undiagnosed.

Tim has volunteered to take a look. I have *cordially* declined his offer.

I'm seeing a specialist soon. And this saga, ongoing, not pretty, accompanied Joe's heart stopping.

Who's got this?

I don't.

I just don't.

16

My Gatsby Green Light
(undated, September 2015)

I'm not in constant pain.

The chemo mostly leaves me in a perpetual state of low-level grossness. I take nausea meds. I do not puke. I take a sleeping pill. I barely sleep. I hate drugs, and I'm on Ambien at night so I feel like an addict.

Right after chemo, my glands seem swollen—but I'm not sure that they really are. I feel weak, really weak. My limbs ache.

I lose my taste for coffee. It comes back before the next round. I persist, drinking coffee every morning nevertheless.

I guess I want to be a coffee-drinker.

The fake breasts are just weird, not right, sort of uncomfortable. But it isn't that they hurt. They're just not *right*. I asked another "survivor" if I'd ever forget that they're there, if I'd lose awareness of these strange things sewn (sewn!) onto my body.

She said that I would not.

What hurts the most doesn't really hurt at all. But it's utterly terrifying.

After chemo, right there in the chemo room, the nurses put this little patch on my stomach—right on the roll of fat some of us have— and this patch has a built-in timer so that it injects an immune-building, get-up-the-white-blood-count medicine into me twenty-four hours after chemo. Automatically!

The needle goes into the fat in the chemo room. A little light blinks in warning, and in two or three minutes the needle goes into my roll of fat with a "pop" that totally scares the hell out of me. And then it's in.

That needle stays in my skin until the time is right: twenty-four hours later. Poised, in my flesh, ready for action. The patch has an adhesive, and a green light flashes to indicate it's working. My fat roll pulsates, my own Gatsby green light.

In twenty-four hours, the meds flow. And then it stings, slightly.

We wait a little bit.

Tim removes the patch (I think the needle recedes or something) before we watch *The Sopranos*. I could do this all myself, but it scares me—like the drains did during those first few weeks post-double mastectomy. (I never clearly wrote about those two gross surgical bulbs that hung from each side of my body and collected disgusting red bloody body fluid that had to be emptied and measured when they got full—Tim changed those too; they were removed before we went to Disney World. I hated them fiercely. This is now us. This is who we now are.)

Everything—from expanding my breasts once a week to waiting for the needle to prick my fat—is low-level, persistent *not-rightness*.

All is not well in the world.

I'm struck, constantly, by how outside the realm of normalcy it is to have one's breasts re-fashioned from silicon and tissue expanders. I want to talk to the plastic surgeon about this, make him divulge his thoughts on the weirdness: His trade? Craft? Vocation?

But he won't have it.

What do you think about all this?

Isn't it weird?

Are we weird here?

My plastic surgeon is uber-professional, a tad detached, kind but not chatty.

So I take his treatments, grateful nonetheless, tissues expanding.

17

Ba-Da-Bing (September 29, 2015)

I really haven't been so hot.

This week, I've thought a lot about revision, reconstruction.

Mostly, of course, what I do as a writer is revise. I turn over a sentence, lifting the words in a phrase, shaking them out like a dusty old rug. The words fly up, like sparks maybe. I catch them before they land, before dust settles, sparks fizzle. I hold those words in the palm of my hand, cradle them really, and put them down delicately, deliberately, brightened, in the proper order (I hope). If you look closely, if you're prone to count syllables or tap out rhythms, you see the words in a sentence spread out like the links in a DNA chain.

In the spirit of revision, I thought I might subtitle my book.

First, I checked out the market—superficially. Obviously, I'll need to denounce my self-imposed ban of the cancer library. But I will not—I repeat, *I will not*—begin identifying myself as a Cancer Survivor. (Cancer Survivor can be a full-time job, I've noticed. Surely, this can't be right.) I do, though, need to read some of the literature. Which is mostly about surviving cancer. Or eating kale. Or staying away from toxic dumps.

Second, I brainstormed potential subtitles. Friends made suggestions. I ignored them.

CANCER, I'LL GIVE YOU ONE YEAR: A NON-INFORMATIVE GUIDE TO BREAST CANCER . . . or

CANCER, I'LL GIVE YOU ONE YEAR: HOW TO GET YOUR BA-DA-BING BOOBIES ON THE HOUSE!

But not: *CANCER, I'LL GIVE YOU ONE YEAR: BUT NOW MY KIDS ARE HIGH-RISK*

My fake breasts are not yet Ba-Da-Bing, but they're not bad.

Granted, you could break open a coconut on them.

Or remember that part in the Bible when Jacob used a stone for a pillow?

I bet he wasn't actually talking about a rock; rather, he was reclining on someone with tissue expanders.

Tim, incidentally, has told me that he, too, is writing a book: *Your Cancer Made Me Fat.*

All of this free food!

I think I've figured out the roles of my doctors, incidentally. My plastic surgeon is the *Whatever Guy.* The oncologist is the *Go-to-the-ER Guy.* This is how it works.

Listen carefully, women. One in eight of you may need to take this to heart.

I go to my plastic surgeon to get my boobs tweaked weekly. This is a conversation we might have:

Me, shirt off, breasts exposed: "I think I'm having heart pains. I'm not sure, but it started last night. Right here." (I put my hand on my chest, far from my heart.)

Plastic Surgeon, gesturing that I should lean back on the table, so he can get this boob-fill going: "*Whatever.*"

Me, leaning back but wondering if my wig is askew—*Might it fall off? Wouldn't that be something?*: "And this breast is bigger than the other. I noticed that. It's way bigger. And I feel like this breast is in my armpit. Like it's *right* in my armpit."

Plastic Surgeon, poking me with the crazy injector thing: "*Whatever.*"

Me, staring off into space, pretending this isn't the weirdest thing in the world: "I'm also not sleeping. How do people sleep? I can't sleep. These breasts are so hard. I'm not sleeping one bit."

Plastic Surgeon, going for the other breast: "*Whatever.*"

He's the *Whatever Guy.*

Then, I go in for chemo—now once a week also. Before every treatment, I see my oncologist. Allow me to begin by saying that my oncologist is a strikingly kind man.

Me, looking pretty damn awesome relative to the other cancer patients around there (I may be shabby as compared to the model crowd in the plastic surgeon's office, but I'm *hot* in oncology!): "I've noticed a little blood on the toilet paper when I, um, have a bowel movement."

Tim, who's there and loves to talk fecal matter: "She's bleeding out her ass."

Oncologist: "Your bloodwork looks great. We'll get you a specialist. But don't hesitate, when things like this happen, to *go to the ER*."

Me, thinking Oh-Dear-Lord-I-Can't-See-Another-Doctor: "I had minor chest pains the other day. I don't think it was a big deal. They stopped after a while."

Oncologist: "If that happens again, *go to the ER*."

Tim, looking to see if there's a fresh pot of coffee in the vicinity: "She's a faker."

Me, forming a little story in my head that I can work on later, one in which this woman gives up her boobs but gains the world: "Do you think it's a problem that I felt this strange swelling rise up from my chest into my neck and ears? It stopped, though—right before my vision got blurry."

Oncologist: "No—but, if it happens again, *go to the ER*."

Tim, getting up because he's ready to be done: "She's a Drama Queen. Best to ignore her."

* * *

And so let me tell you how chemo has pushed me into menopause: forty-five and it's over!

Ba-da-bing!

I don't really care that I'm in menopause, because we're done with kids, my identity as a woman isn't tied up in my menstrual cycle like it is in my breasts, and we could cash in on the no-birth-control bit, which will be handy when we have sex once a year on Valentine's Day.

But menopause is *happening*!

OK, you hear a lot about these hot flashes, but what the fuck are they?

I'm here to tell you: That's just what they are. *Hot flashes*. Suddenly, wherever you are, whatever you're doing, you begin to radiate heat. You break out into a sweat. The sweat drips off your temples, off the bridge of your nose. Your breasts, fake or not, collect moisture underneath them. If you're wearing a wig, you're in trouble because it feels like the cat is napping on your head. If you're trying to sleep, forget it. You'll whip the sheets off to cool down. Then, later, you might get cold, so you'll pull the sheets back on. But then you'll get hot again. This will go on all night. Forget contact with another human being, because people are space heaters.

I don't think Tim really got it until we went to the Apple Store this past weekend to—finally!—get me a new laptop.

The young Genius (they call those techie kids *geniuses*) was doing very well in pretending that I wasn't an idiot when I asked things like, "I can save documents with this, right?"

70

We were already a little class-conscious in the Scottsdale Quarter because we're poor and I was wearing yoga pants.

But then, then, *the hot flash*: The sweat started cascading down me. Rolling off my face. Streaking my cheeks.

I picked a laptop and admitted to the Genius that I was ACTUALLY A COLLEGE PROFESSOR.

The Genius said, "May I see your faculty ID, so I can offer you a teacher's discount?"

I was *pouring* sweat. I tried to find my faculty ID in my purse. Gum wrappers, shopping lists, Post-its, random programs from events held six months ago popped out. A tampon fell on the floor (apparently, I used to carry them around). Tim wanted to help. "Let me help," he said.

I didn't need help. "I'm fine." I knew my ID was in there. I'd find it in a second.

Just give me a damn minute.

Give me one fucking minute.

Me, wild-eyed, sweating, glowing. Tim, reaching for my purse like he knows where everything is.

Back the hell off, people!

The Genius stepped away, and Tim said, "Jen, you're really sweating."

"I am?"

I think he thought I was nervous about spending a million bucks on a Mac, about being surrounded by all those rich people, about wearing my ripped underwear in this neighborhood.

But the truth is that I didn't give a shit about any of those things: It was a hot flash!

The Genius was a little intimidating, but I'm sure I could teach him a thing or two about the Oxford comma.

The reality is that menopause had hit.

Hard.

I've been sad lately. Mostly about my marriage, about the toll cancer is taking.

Let's move on. Hot flashes to marriage. Why not? It's the end of September, the heart of chemo, I am bald and breastless.

I love the guy, my husband. He's usually nice to me (except sometimes when he's a total asshole). We talk about crazy stuff. We've grown into each other. He says funny things. When he walks past an open window, he says, "What if I was doing something weird?" When he's gone, I miss him.

But we're out of sync. I'm driving him crazy. He's tired of my cancer, its hold on me. I'm sick of his routines, their demands. We're past the desperation of the moment; we're into the commitment, the wait, the endurance. There's revision now, reconstruction. We will make it; I know this. *But how will we be when this is over?*

And does it really end?

I asked him one night, "Do you think we'll bounce back?" *To our usual happy-go-lucky, thrilled-to-be-together selves?*

"Yeah," he said, like he meant it. *Did he mean it?*

But I wonder: *How far does this revision, this reconstruction go? Where will it take us? Will the parts, when they settle, make sense?*

Ba-Da-Bing?

And it's not easy. I'm telling you: my chest hurts. My heart. It may be my heart. I'm pretty sure it's my heart.

18

I'm on Drugs (October 1, 2015)

I'm writing this to see if I can, after taking ten milligrams of Ambien last night (I've been taking five, and it doesn't work). I'm giving myself till 9 a.m. only. So bear with me. I want to see if I can still write.

I woke at 4:30 a.m.—or, at least, I got out of bed at 4:30 a.m.—but I was fuzzy. I think I was A-OK by 5:15.

Yesterday: Chemo Day.

First, I taught, only taking a quick moment to have a hot flash during my second class. I had to tell them, since I suddenly broke out into a sweat while discussing the text. "Guys, I'm going through menopause—you know what that is?—and I'm having a hot flash. Hold tight," I told my class, which largely consisted of male athletes. They looked on in wonder.

Next, I headed home, texting Tim. He takes the day off on Chemo Days. Our routine is to go out for a very cheap lunch and then head over for the good time.

Well, we got into a fight over text. I'm not going to tell you about what we were fighting about, since it's one of our usual fights and I'll probably fictionalize it later, making him look like a complete mofo and making me look like the clear victor. Believe me, too, I will play the Cancer Card in my rendition, which will only make Tim look worse.

We "resolved" it (*buried it under the rug*). We met at the house and ate McDonald's in the car on the way to chemo.

Then, I saw my oncologist.

"Incessant hot flashes," I said, my mouth gaping. I pointed at my tonsils and mouthed, *Water*.

I have to avoid estrogen from here on out because it feeds my kind of cancer (estrogen-positive). So, I'm stuck with the hot flashes. "There's a med for them, but it's an antidepressant," the oncologist said.

And here's my official word on antidepressants. I will read all hate mail. *I don't do them.*

For one reason only: I'm a *writer.*

I have tossed this around with many fine psychiatrists and doctors and artists. Most of them say that I'm wrong. I will admit this from the onset.

Here's some over-the-top honesty. I'd probably qualify for mild—*pretty mild*—clinical depression. But, damn it, I'll be depressed. I'll take my sorrows, my heavy heart, my suspicion that the world is fucked. I simply cannot take something that will mess with my brain chemistry and possibly affect my ability to write.

I guess I make an exception for coffee.

Don't tell me the other ways I volitionally alter my brain chemistry. Hold your tongue!

But I want to be clear—and now I'm talking to all you Self-Righteous-Terribly-Old-School-Types-Who-Think-No-One-Should-Take-Antidepressants. First, you don't know what you're talking about. You're wrong. Second, some people really need them. There are legitimate chemical imbalances. I believe in antidepressants. I think it's super naïve to suggest that people with these imbalances can manage them if they tried, prayed, sought God.

I'm not even sure that I would resist for myself if my depression weren't so low-level. (I get a little too sad, then angry, followed by cussing.)

Bottom line: *Hello, hot flashes!*

I guess you guys can stick around.

I headed into the chemo room, following our hot flash consultation. New chemo meds! I'm through the worst of it! But they started me off with fifty milligrams of Benadryl to ward off nausea.

That's just not gonna work for me.

I'd rather vomit, thank you very much.

Not only could I not read which I really wanted to do, but I also couldn't get comfortable or fall asleep. So, I just fidgeted and—this is true—went to the bathroom about six times.

But there's more. Thinking that I might fall asleep, I pulled out my contacts without looking in a mirror, which rendered me very impaired. But at least I wouldn't fall asleep in my contacts.

Though I never fell asleep.

So I was just blind.

(And I got unreasonably sad, then pretty angry, followed by much cussing.)

Tim was incredibly busy playing Sudoku, but I didn't want to hear him say a word anyway. I just stumbled blindly into the chemo room toilet to pee half-a-dozen times. The nurses, who are awesome, agreed to cut my dose to twenty-five milligrams of Benadryl next time. I asked them to give me only a quarter of it. They said they would on the third visit.

I need to read books while getting chemo. No antidepressants, no Benadryl.

We finished up for the day, I peed some more, and we headed to the car—me holding onto Tim since I couldn't see and the Arizona sun was blinding at 4:45 p.m. *The car battery was dead!* Would you believe it? Tim called AAA, and I went back inside to sit in the waiting room, cancered out and blind.

Seriously!

I had just had chemo, I was tweaking on Benadryl, and I couldn't see a thing.

The AAA guy showed. What happened next is something I need to be careful about. The guy showed up in the time frame promised. He did his job fine. I wouldn't want him to lose his job, and he's probably going to at some point soon.

Poor, poor guy.

Tim texted me to come out to the parking lot—even though I was blind. I did. The guy—uber-friendly—was behaving a little maniacally. He brought me water, since Tim had told AAA that they needed to hurry their asses up because his wife had just had chemo. The guy was kind, and professional—more or less. Just crazy talkative.

Tim typed something on his phone and showed it to me: *drugs.*

We don't really know, of course. There was no real evidence. But I gotta tell you this: *My unpublished novel, which you are not getting a free copy of, is about bath salt addiction. So, this isn't something entirely foreign to me or to Tim.*

We know the signs.

Why didn't we freak out when he was installing a new battery in our car?

Because we knew perfectly well that he could do it. These guys love the miniscule detail work involved in bolts and wires. They do fuck up, no doubt. But it would be OK. Plus, Tim was right there. And I was blind and drugged out myself—so best to just go with it.

The guy finished, and the car worked fine.

Got home about 6:30 p.m.!

I'm sad for this AAA guy. By the time this book is published, he'll have lost his job (and he has three kids), or he'll be clean.

I gave myself till 9 a.m. It's 9:15. Did the ten milligrams of Ambien I took last night get out of my system? Am I writing OK?

19

Bombshell (October 9, 2015)

Tim woke up saying, "We won't sue."

So much for the book he says he's writing, which had almost undergone a title change: *Your Cancer Made Me Fat . . . and Rich.*

We won't pursue a malpractice case. There will be no money. I will die a pauper.

* * *

Bombshell yesterday—which could possibly be construed as good news (I guess), but has legal ramifications. I don't know if I should talk about it. My lawyer wants me to shut up.

My lawyer!

I get it.

But there's this other, far more driven, part of me that wants to write it all down immediately, with complete candor, legality be damned.

Tim doesn't entirely get my compulsion, my impatience for revelation— *Can't I wait a bit?*—but he's also accustomed to my pursuits.

I waited till we decided not to sue anyone.

We're not suing anyone.

There.

That's done.

It's over.

I can talk.

Allow me to begin this saga with a caveat: I'm a fiction writer. I've published two books of fiction. I've never published a book of nonfiction. I may be making this up.

Writers are liars?

I received news yesterday.

Here are the undisputed facts:

I've been in touch with a lawyer since early on, because I actually found a small lump by my right nipple in October 2014. It felt like a disgusting hard zit.

Have I written the word *nipple* before?

(I don't like saying *nipple*. I kinda want to giggle into my arm or cover my mouth with my hand. *Nipple nipple nipple!*

I had a mammogram and an ultrasound in October 2014, after discovering the lump.

Tim was there that day. We were nervous. After the ultrasound, we were told it was nothing, one of those cyst-things women get. No biopsy was ordered. And since I have—or *had*—dense breasts, the cyst—much like a zit—would break up on its own. Case closed. I win.

We sighed in relief, and promptly went out for lunch at Dickey's BBQ. Dickey's was so great that we decided to cater our Thanksgiving dinner from there, much to the polite chagrin of my mom and probably Tim's parents, too—they found catered barbecue for Thanksgiving to be unorthodox and a little gauche.

But what the hell?

I didn't have cancer!

October 2014 cancer scare in the bag.

Cancer diagnosis in June 2015. Right breast.

* * *

More than a few people, but especially my sister-in-law, who was the most convincing, told me to talk to a lawyer about medical malpractice.

Did the radiologist miss something in October 2014?

Why wasn't a biopsy ordered?

Would treatment have differed had it been done?

Would I, had cancer been diagnosed then, have only needed a lumpectomy rather than a mastectomy?

Would chemo have been necessary?

What kind of chemo?

Would it have been a "lighter" regimen?

Would I have needed radiation?

What kind, if any, reconstruction would have been necessary?

And maybe most importantly: *Would it have made it to my lymph nodes?*

Tim and I got in touch with medical malpractice lawyers—a difficult field because it's expensive and doctors do not like to testify against other doctors. As of today, I also learned that mammography is an especially problematic field, and it's tough to say what's worthy of attention and what's not. I quietly went back to my radiologist and gathered my records and films, which spanned back a few years.

Well, the lawyers got an expert opinion, who specialized in dense breast mammography.

Here's the bombshell, according to one expert: *A mistake was made. I've had breast cancer since June 2014.*

JUNE 2014!

* * *

In the summer of 2014, we took a road trip to Utah, Colorado, and New Mexico. We stayed with my aunt and uncle in Denver. I had a reading for *Love Slave* at BookBar, and Tim and I had dinner with my editor.

It was a great trip, even though I made Wendy walk through the Arches National Park till she puked, thereby ruining Utah forever for her. We loved Denver. We loved Santa Fe. I thought Utah was crazy beautiful.

Cancer the whole time!

* * *

I had had a routine mammogram in June 2014—before this trip. The mammogram had come back as normal. The films were shown to the expert.

At that point, according to this one expert, *I already had Stage 2A breast cancer.* There were two tumors, and they were too far apart for a lumpectomy, so even at that point, I was still only a candidate for a mastectomy.

That I would still need a mastectomy, rather than a lumpectomy, is very important. In the legal world, a malpractice case isn't wise: *Though the cancer was already there, the treatment would have been the same.*

This is probably—*probably*—not a winnable case. As long as the treatment would have been the same.

The good news is that it only went from Stage 2A to Stage 2B.

Yay!

Let's be careful here: *It's one opinion.*

Dr. Radiologist, I am not going to sue you.

I understand that hindsight is twenty/twenty.

I understand that doctors make difficult decisions, and not all decisions are due to negligence.

I am contemplating the possibility of negligence.

Friends, we tossed it around all day, all night. Tim and I were at odds. The lawyer tried to keep it real. We spoke on the phone numerous times. "Unless your treatment would've been different, there is no case," the lawyer repeated. I would be looking at an arduous, expensive, stressful legal battle that could be lost or dropped, which happens a lot. "And your cancer wouldn't go away as a result."

Tim came home from work early, stressed out, and he immediately wrote something:

> For the most part, I think the issue of there being a case hinges on how we delineate "treatment." When the expert says "treatment would not have changed," I don't know if she is speaking as a surgeon, an oncologist, or a radiologist. I think this matters a great deal. When we met with our oncologist prior to surgery, he was in agreement that the cancer was too invasive and required a mastectomy. He was not 100 percent sure chemo would be required, though. A lot depended on the lymph node biopsy—although again, he was inclined towards chemo regardless of what the lymph node biopsy showed. If he were to have examined you in June 2014, I am doubtful he would have proceeded in exactly the same way. In fact, I would be surprised if the treatment wouldn't have been radically different. There might have been the treatment with Tamoxifen to shrink one or both of the tumors, and to make a call on lumpectomy vs. mastectomy based on that.
>
> The chemotherapy is, by far, the worst part of this whole thing. That is where the needless suffering is coming from. This could be itemized for sure but, in the very least, and apart from any punitive damages, you lost the ability to work full time while I am burning through all my sick and vacation time. Then there are the medical expenses associated with the chemo regimen. However, I doubt that sum is significant enough to cover the trial and make it worth pursuing. So the punitive element would have to be defined here, but only what comes from the potentially needless chemotherapy.
>
> Then there is the likely fact that in 2014, the cancer would not have made it into the lymph nodes. Therefore, a lymph node biopsy would not have been performed (most likely) and you wouldn't have the rest of your life affected by damage to the lymph ducts that occur during that biopsy.
>
> Then there is radiation part. We don't even know the misery that comes from that yet, but lifelong scar tissue and hardening

are not uncommon. Probably plenty of expense from this as well. Most likely, this would not be indicated either had we caught it in 2014.

Then there is the metastatic risk. One node was positive. There is good reason to expect the prognosis would have been more sure had it never made it to the lymph nodes. All we know is that it was allowed enough time to metastasize to the lymph node.

Tim's job is in cancer, folks.

I cannot get compensated for many things in a medical malpractice case. We postponed getting a dog. I look like a zombie from *The Walking Dead*, a Baby Orangutan in the zoo. Our marriage has been taxed. I'm depressed often enough, my temper is short, and I worry if we'll ever really recover from this. We hate our kitchen sink. We didn't fix the blinds in the house. We didn't re-carpet one of the bedrooms. We pay a million co-pays. I'm the big anti-drug advocate here, and I'm on narcotics.

None of this is eligible for legal damages.

I'm not interested in fighting a lengthy case, which will stress out my family, not take away my cancer, and cost a lot of money.

Dr. Radiologist, you are not responsible for my cancer.

I am not saying you are.

One thing my lawyer said to me—and I might add that we're closely philosophically aligned on things—"You don't want to get into the revenge business."

* * *

Dr. Radiologist, here are some random cancer things for this October.

I suspect my eyelashes are falling out.

Enough can't be said about the people who show up willing to help. It's really hard to grasp such grace. Women armed with pesto, Five Guys' gift cards. We eat cups of Cold Stone. Our bread is freshly made, the loaves unsliced. Tim's work sends home salmon with lemon wedges, scalloped potatoes in someone's good dishes, a melon and bacon and feta cheese salad we eat in slow bites. Moms drive my kids to school, take them home for playdates for long stretches of time on quiet Sunday afternoons, school nights, too.

I may try to slip into bed tonight with my sexy husband with whom I barely have sex. Perhaps I'll put a paper bag over my head, somehow camouflage my chemo port, and make a move on him. *Perhaps . . . .*

* * *

Dr. Radiologist, I was made for cancer.

What I lack in sleep, I make up for in reading and writing. Professorial of course, unpaid for sure. I write an envious amount. Reading Philip Roth, MLK, Chimamanda Ngozi Adichie, Harper Lee!

I've admitted something to Tim, but maybe it sounds nuts: "If I knew I'd live through this, if I knew I wouldn't die, this cancer thing is OK."

It's fine with me. I'm—dare I say it?—even good. As a writer, I'm good with experiencing it. The double mastectomy, the chemo, the reconstruction. I'll take it all, even the part where I have no breasts. Just to *experience* it. Even though I've said so many times that I want a normal life, I really don't want a normal life.

Yes, I was made for cancer.

Let us not speak of how I was made for suffering.

* * *

Dr. Radiologist, yesterday, one of my best friends from college visited.

And we had fun with my body parts.

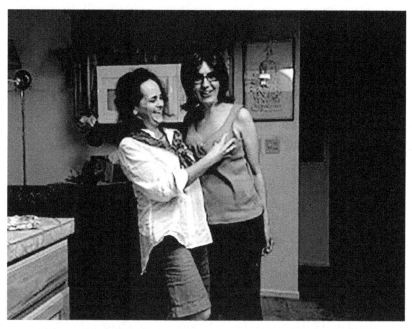

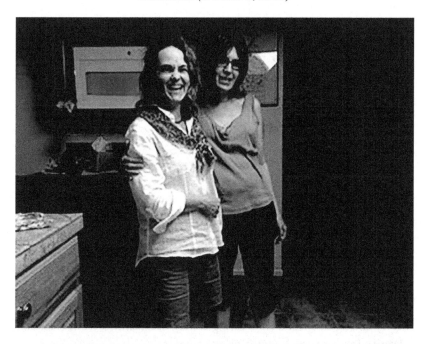

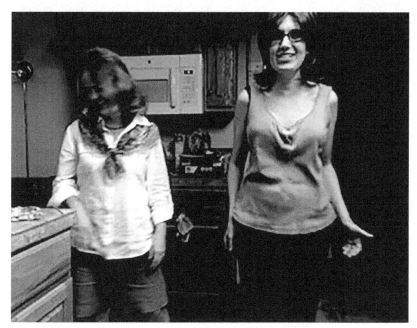

Photos by Tim Bell.

20

No Light, No Light (October 14, 2015)

Mom, before you go any further, do not go nuts on me over the title of this chapter. It's a song by Florence + The Machine whose concert I just missed, thereby ending an era and announcing, loudly, decadently, lavishly (Florence is lavish), *Jennifer needs to stay home after dark*.

Well, storytelling is the real topic here: the heart of story, the truth of it.

First, a disturbing tale about where the light don't shine.

No light, no light.

I finally got an appointment with the GI (gastrointestinal doc) about the ... *you know*. It's been a little over a month of ... *you know*. Did someone say *anal fissure*?

(Florence + The Machine is a no-go, but an anal probe is happening— this is the "new" me, cancered up in 2015.)

I waited fifty minutes to see him. Having finished my novel, I was about to complain. There's only so much time you can happily spend on your smart phone.

Then, he walks in. I almost got up right there and left. Not because he kept me waiting for fifty minutes—*forget that*—but because he was this *totally hot guy in his mid-twenties!*

He must've finished his residency yesterday.

Thanks, but no thanks.

So what if my ass is bleeding?

Cancer-schmancer!

See you later, Hot Doc!

But I stayed.

Keep in mind that I had just answered the question on his paperwork about whether or not I was sexually active by saying, "Theoretically." And I had felt pretty damn clever about it too. *Theoretically! Ha! Aren't I funny? Theoretically!*

I sat still, taking my own pulse, while he whispered (he really did have this whisper of a deep voice), "We should schedule your colonoscopy for next Tuesday."

Next Tuesday: *I'm going under, and he's going in.*

I was so mesmerized by his hotness that I forgot to mention that my oncologist said something about nothing invasive during chemo. My guess is that an anal probe is invasive.

See you Tuesday, Hot Doc!

A friend suggested that I take a selfie with him.

I bet the rest of you are wondering about my in-your-face ogling of this six-foot-*plus* doctor, *who was also dark and handsome*—since I'm married, and sexually active (theoretically!). Do we have an open marriage like Will and Jada?

Hell, no.

I've seen Tim jealous exactly two times, and both instances were completely absurd. I could go away for the weekend with the Butt Doctor, and Tim would just want to make sure he had enough cereal and raisins till I got home. He might want to know if I'd be back in time for *The Walking Dead* on Sunday. Both instances of jealousy on his part were early in our marriage. Once, he expressed jealousy over Rob, the *fictional* character in my novel, *Love Slave*. And, on another occasion, he admitted to being jealous of my Bono poster. That's right. *Once, he was jealous of a made-up guy, and another time, he was jealous of a piece of paper.* (So, moms, this is like being jealous of Flat Stanley.)

Other than that, *nothing*.

You can look at his lack of jealousy in two ways: Perhaps this says something profound about who he is as a man, his character, his understanding of love, *blah blah blah*—or it says something about me: *Full of hot air. And he knows it.*

Which might be expelled against my wishes in the hot doc's face during the anal probe on Tuesday.

I, on the other hand, am an extremely jealous woman. It's not pretty. Don't get me started. Right now, it's Lana Del Ray. *Skank.*

Lana, I'm so sorry. Really, I have nothing against you whatsoever except for the fact that you seem to have some sort of gross affiliation with James Franco, who might love himself a bit too much, as evidenced in his selfie-obsession, though I am possibly just jealous of him myself since he is kinda overly talented with his spontaneous advanced degrees and books of both poetry and prose and Faulkner film adaptations and shit. (I saw *The Interview*, buddy.) I don't know, Lana, if you're a skank or not and, anyway, an editor will edit this out—they won't let it go to print—*so don't worry.* I won't be allowed to call you a skank, even though I think (just a little) your music is kinda all surface and no substance. I guess I'm thinking you've got that sensuality thing going like Tori Amos did back in the day, *that sensuality thing that fools horny guys*—but, *unlike* Tori, you may lack the talent. *You're no Tori Amos, Lana.* You can fool the guys because *they're guys,* but you're not gonna fool the women.

You. Will. Not. Fool. The. Women.

Why am I ripping on Lana Del Ray? She'll freakin' sue me! (*Lana, don't sue me!* I don't have any breasts, for God's sake! My eyelashes are falling out! You wouldn't, would you? You're not a skank! You're not!)

For the record, Lana Del Ray is not a skank!

This goes back to Tim! *It's his fault.* I know *love is not jealous,* and all that, but C'MON!

At any rate, I better cover my ass—*again with the ass-talk!*—by saying something nice about celebrities I know nothing about. *Tina Fey, I wish we were friends. Mindy Kaling, you go girl! Bono, I do love you! I really do!*

Lana, it's Tim's fault.

* * *

Back to storytelling. Since I'm writing a book in real-time, I spent a few hours (minutes) looking at the cancer book market. It turns out that not only do one in eight women get breast cancer, *but all eight of them write books about* it.

I've FINALLY, CRAZILY got the market cornered, however! I'm not so sure there are ANY cancer books like mine. The others all fulfill a function that I just don't: *They provide helpful information.*

My book will clearly not help you.

But what I seem to do—or be willing to do—is expose myself for the sake of the narrative. People often say that my writing is honest, and I'm very flattered by this (believe me), but I think it's more accurate to say that I'll put myself out there for the sake of narrative, of storytelling.

The other books are about cancer. My book is about story.

I'm interested in literary nonfiction!

I don't even care about the cancer!

(Sometimes, I think to myself—when I'm reading the work of others, *Why so guarded? What are you protecting?*)

I guess this is an admission right here, a philosophy on literary nonfiction: It's self-centered. It's true—but make no mistake about it: It's crafted truth.

I love that thing I just wrote: *Literary nonfiction is crafted truth!*

Man, who came up with that?

Did I?

(I seriously doubt it. I probably read it somewhere. Wait. Bruce Ballenger wrote *Crafting Truth* in 2010 and Louise Spence and Vinicius Navarro wrote *Crafting Truth: Documentary Form and Meaning*, also in 2010. I didn't read either, which probably means that I, as a creative writing prof, just heard it somewhere and stole it. You know what Andy Warhol said, right? Whoops. Pablo Picasso. Picasso said, "[G]ood artists borrow, great artists steal." Then, King Solomon said in Ecclesiastes that there's nothing new under the sun. And I remember being profoundly moved during the *Achtung Baby/Zooropa* stage, when Bono sang, "Every artist is a cannibal / every poet is a thief / all kill for inspiration / and then sing about their grief." But, somehow, I'm feeling like Andy Warhol fits into this crafted truth bit. Maybe Andy Warhol really said *THAT*? I don't know, but you get the point. I actually really believe this shit. Like, perhaps, two big principles or ideas of my own creative writing aesthetic are a belief in redemptive endings and a belief that artists are cannibals. For the greater good. And, usually or hopefully, it's that artists will eat *themselves* alive for the greater good? Oh, wait. I'm writing a book on cancer . . . .)

Well, one more thing. The Florence + The Machine concert I didn't go to last night.

Why is this so important to me?

I bought tickets with a friend right before the diagnosis. Once the cancer life kicked in, I thought I'd still go. Why not?

But on this previous Saturday night, around 8 or 9 p.m.—when I was in full-fledged zombie-mode—I turned to Tim, and asked, "What am I *thinking*? I *can't* go to Florence + The Machine!" It hit me: I'm not able to converse after dark, I no longer sleep, I teach in the morning, I have chemo the day after the concert, I'm having hot flashes every three minutes, there's a dead animal on my head, and, well, *I'm scared.*

I bailed on my friend and dumped the tickets.

And so ends my rock n' roll era: You don't get closure with cancer.

So much for the redemptive end?

Try weaving a strong narrative out of this.

You will die first.

* * *

In truth, my rock n' roll era ended this spring.

I can't really talk about it, because I'm unreasonably upset by the experience. *OK, I'll talk about it.*

We took the kids to see U2 in May 2015—my little familial fantasy of passing the torch—and it was a colossal bust.

We left because it was too loud and it hurt their ears. Tim took Wendy out after three songs. THREE songs. I followed with Melody shortly thereafter (she was begging to go). We found our car, which we had parked illegally, and went home. And there ends the U2 Saga!

My sweet Wendy, now, NOW, post-diagnosis, feels badly about how U2 sucked for me. She got a little sad when I told her that I couldn't make it to Florence.

She asked, "Will you see Florence + The Machine another time?"

I said, "Probably not." I was just being honest. "But I'll probably see U2 again. Don't worry about it."

She recently said, "I wish U2 would come back so I could make it up to you."

So, today, now about an hour away from chemo, I say to you that I hope to write an unguarded cancer story—not about malignant tumors, but about antiheroes and cannibals. Antiheroes who do not always rise above the situation and pontificate sanctimoniously on inner beauty. Cannibals with the kind of invasive cancer that taints body, taints soul—and, still, they eat themselves alive, feeding on the tainted meat.

People who just wanted to go hear Florence + The Machine sing that one song.

You want a revelation? You want a resolution?
It's a conversation I just can't have tonight.

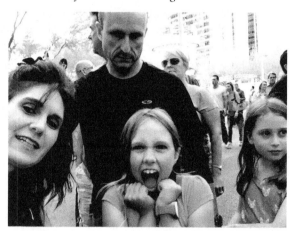

The official end of my rock n' roll era: Family photo at U2 concert on May 23, 2015 (about one month before diagnosis): *Bust.* Photo by the author.

21

Up Yours! (October 19, 2015)

W ell, *that* was fun.

This will be a short chapter because—really—even I might draw the line here.

Today, I had a colonoscopy and an upper endoscopy. Finally, after maybe more than a month of what we might politely call "rectal bleeding," I saw the doctor (who proved to be a hottie) and scheduled this outpatient procedure. I suspected the blood was an effect of chemo, but everyone was on red alert: *Perhaps it was colon cancer.*

The hot doctor troubled me the most, and I couldn't exactly complain to my oncologist—the recipient of all medical complaints—that the doctor he sent me to was too attractive to do an anal probe. ("Can you refer me to an uglier doctor?")

When I envisioned it, I was very unhappy: One probe in the butt, one probe in the mouth, me out cold, probably in a very unflattering fetal position, wigless (because would they let me wear it in a supposedly sterile environment or, if they did, would it accidentally slip and they'd try to fix it, but they wouldn't really be able to—so I'd either wake with it absurdly askew or looking like my old Baby Orangutan-self?). This was not a pretty picture.

Actually, I wore my skullcap. Which isn't any better. A cross between me *Going Gangster* and me *Going Holocaust.*

The night before the probe is not fun.

First, one fasts with a liquid diet. No cream in my coffee. I drank four cups of chicken broth, which I can't recommend.

Then, one drinks this bizarre prescription brew whose aim it is to, um, clear you out. *Which it does. All night long. Maybe sixteen times.*

I thought they were joking.

They were not.

* * *

And just because you don't have cancer, do not assume you're safe. They recommend yearly colonoscopies for everyone after the age of fifty (this might be changing). But you are safe from other things. I had to go in for immune-boosting shots on Friday and Monday (with more bloodwork on Monday).

The procedure itself was OK. They did make me take a surprise pregnancy test, and Tim and I had to muffle our boisterous laughter.

Then, the nurse missed my vein when she inserted the IV, and that hurt.

But another nurse was a big fan of *The Walking Dead*, and she was totally caught up—so we immediately launched into a serious discussion on Carol and Carl and how Morgan needs to get his shit together. When that nurse left, Tim whispered, "You asked the nurse the same question twice."

"How did she respond?" I asked.

"She graciously answered twice."

What did I say about nurses?

Didn't I tell you?

I know I said something.

Is there an index in this book?

Can you look it up?

Hardest working people out there.

Did I say that twice?

As for the hot doctor, Tim said, "He really wasn't all that hot."

(*He was.*)

I only saw him for five minutes: two and a half minutes before the procedure and two and a half minutes after the procedure.

Doctors! Even the hot ones!

* * *

It was a hemorrhoid.

Bullhorn, please: *Jennifer Spiegel has a hemorrhoid!*

Allow me to quote myself: *I'm OK with all of this, if I live through it.*

This is an opportunity. *An emersion experience.*

I thought about this for a fleeting moment today, sitting in this special chair in my two gowns (one like a jacket open in the front, one like a smock open in the back, buck naked underneath), waiting for my port to get poked, seeing Tim dressed all "normal" nearby. This was, in only a few short months, not all that weird for us. *I am sick, and we are used to it.* I am now an ailment, propelled from procedure to procedure, just like that one relative you have who always needs to be tested or who always has a racing heart: *I am her.* On that chair, I looked at Tim and wondered if I had become to him that one relative who needs first a colonoscopy and then a little radiation, first one test and then another.

I'm only interested in a temporary emersion experience.

22

The Novelty of Cancer (October 28, 2015)

My cancer is getting tiresome, yes? My family is tired; I see it clearly in their posture, their faces. The drag of it, the *can't we talk about something else* of it. I'm weary, too—from my place "in the thick of it." Something like eight chemo sessions left? I'm sick of my wig—now unflattering, now frizzed (why didn't I go with the other one?), sick of my routine, of anxiety, of fake breasts. The novelty is gone.

In November, the only thing I have planned are weekly chemo sessions, the resumption of the breast "fills" to make it to my coveted C-cups, maybe having a talk with my plastic surgeon about tattoos, and probably the further loss of my eyelashes (and eyebrows, too!). Perhaps there will be sex, but we can skip it for the sake of maintaining mystery. I might eat turkey on Thanksgiving, and—at that point—I really, really need to meditate on gratitude. But I'm thinking that I'll take November off to finish (I hope!) my unintentionally ironically titled novel, *And So We Die, Having First Slept.*

Who thought that one up?

I did a little novel-tweaking yesterday, and I found this odd, lovely line: *Her life had been set up to die, to die a beautiful death.*

Gotta wonder about this book.

Well, a word on the tattoo business. The thought occurred to me—this idea of opting out of nipple reconstruction (*nipple nipple nipple*), which sounds a little weird to me—and getting some big tattoos instead. The thing about nipple reconstruction is that it says *I'm a fake nipple* all over. Nipple reconstruction announces its own lie.

A tattoo says, *Fuck, Yeah.*

I wasn't rock 'n' roll enough to walk around bald. I liked the idea of non-conformity, of defiance, of brazen baldness. But, at the end of the day, I wanted anonymity. I didn't want to hand out cancer announcement cards.

But I'm rock 'n' roll enough to tattoo my breasts.

Tim, incidentally, says he'll get a matching tattoo.

* * *

I'll tell you some other stuff, depressing stuff. *The acuteness of my fragility is pressing,* and—I'm afraid—this kind of pressing is an alienated, private kind. Those you love are just not in it with you.

There was yet another suggestion that I go on an antidepressant. And, once again, I refused. I suppose that this must be part of my book.

What's a memoir if not unflattering in its fullness?

I flat-out refused, and I will continue to do so.

But the truth is I'm no picnic to be around.

Right now, all I can say to those I shit on is this: *I'm sorry.*

Who will survive this with me? Who will stick it out? Will I? Am I too short-sighted to make it through a little cancer?

Here I am now, *depressed.*

This is how it goes: I feel a solid kind of sadness that maybe floats overhead like an odor—the scent of someone else's house that one recognizes but doesn't think about—and it wafts by, sometimes not present, sometimes very present. I work right through it; actually, I *really* work through it. *I go all kamikaze on it.* I put away the dishes, grade the papers, march around the house like a Nazi, whip my world into shape. Even following chemo, I get my to-do list done, damn it. And, if need be, I repress the sorrow. I'm very capable of not acting depressed. So what does that say? What does it mean if one can control one's response to the acuteness of fragility?

Externally?

But not internally?

I realized, early on—not now, but at other times in my life—that my writing is still intact when I'm low. This realization was gold, a blessing, a kind of redemption. What had I been given? How would I use it?

To those who suffer my storm, *I'm sorry again.*

I'm choosing to keep my writing intact, though: no antidepressants.

Cancer, I'll give you one year.

I cannot give you the one thing I'm good at, though.

The writing is not for you.

Listen, I'm OK.

I buckle down in times like these. I get to work.
Did you know we're so fragile?
Did you?

23

Mom Can't Die (November 1, 2015)

First, it's simple.
Who would wash the dishes?
Who would feed the cats?
Who would keep up with immunizations?
Make dentist appointments?
Wash spills off counters, pick up used napkins from the floor?
Clean socks, underwear, school clothes?
Monitor growing feet, buy new shoes?
So many new shoes—.
Sign homework folders, schedule the piano teacher, pour cups of milk?
Get up, no matter what, do it, just do it, sleepless, ill?
Who will micromanage, helicopter, inflict lifelong scars only a mother
can inflict?
Who will be there five minutes early *every single time*?

Then, it's complicated.
Who will say *No*?
Who will say *You're going to break your neck if you do that*?
Who will say *You make a choice, every day you make a choice*?
Who will say *There's suffering*?
Who will say *Make the right choice*?
Who will look in eyes, look at faces, measure woes, count hurts?
Who will hold them?

Who will be brazen enough to say *This is the truth, I am telling you the*
truth?
Who will apologize, parse life, paint it pretty, reveal the ugly,
dole out treasure?

Mom is Big Brother,
Mom is the Committee for Truth and Reconciliation,
The FBI, the CIA, the Executive Branch,
The House of Representatives, the Judiciary
The World Health Organization,
And Amnesty International.

Mom can't die.
That's just it.
Mom can't die.

24

You Already Know About the Fear of Death (November 2015)

Hot Flash, O Hot Flash, Are You Kidding Me?
Hot Flash, O Hot Flash, Make Up Your Fucking Mind.

Two poem titles for unwritten verse,
witty, obscene, F-bomb abuse.
On the easy stuff, the slapstick stuff:
There's the part where I rip off my wig,
in a violent gesture: cartoonish,
the sweat rolling, rolling
cascading, cascading.
There's the part where I whip off the quilt,
more violence—so much violence!
The fan overhead, spinning slowly, leaving me naked in a
wet sheen:
irresistible in my zombie 'do.

But do you know this other part?—
you already know about the Fear of Death—
do you sense this other part?
This new Gnosticism, this new Stoicism—
do you understand the dissociation from one's body?
One's own Art Project
stitched into one's own flesh

so close to the heart, the cave of the chest.
(Do you remember Plato's *Allegory of the Cave*?
The types and shadows? The real and the unreal?
All that talk about shadows?)
This is not quite asceticism, not really hatred either.

So take a gander—just gawk!—
it's not me anymore.

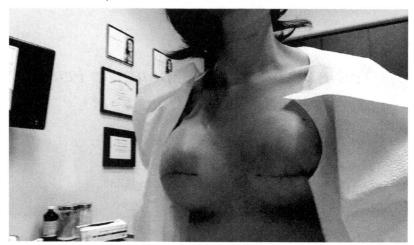

Photo by the author.

25

Snickers (December 1, 2015)

That poem? They're part of my personal art project, definitely desexualized, disassociated.

But who has time for poetry? For art?

We got a freakin' puppy. Snickers. I don't know what we were thinking.

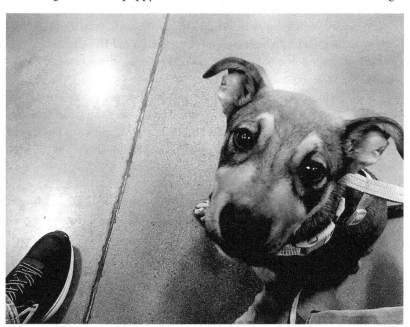

Photo by the author.

I'm regretting it, but we'll push forward, as we've done with many other things in our lives that worked out eventually. The story behind our plunge is probably boring, but not really. We've wanted a dog—a labrador retriever or golden retriever mix—for a very long time (or they all did), and the plan was to get one at the end of the summer of 2015, post-move and post-Disney Extravaganza.

Then, cancer happened.

So we told the kids, "We have to wait."

Till when? After chemo? After radiation? After my boobs, my art project? When? When? *When?*

And so we just did it, our Black Friday binge. We bought a puppy. I'm sure it was ultimately my fault, my call. During the last round of chemo on Wednesday (three treatments left), I looked up Lab rescue websites on my phone, thereby launching the family into dog chaos. By Wednesday night, the poor children were all over the internet, searching for rescue dogs. By Thanksgiving, the house was virtually in a tailspin, no pun intended, or—if intended—only a little intended.

What did we want? Why, high-energy, big breeds only, of course!

By Friday, we had a "lab." Does that look like a labrador retriever to you? I think not.

A twenty-something year-old girl in short-shorts, heavily black eye-lined eyes, long Joni Mitchell hair, and something a tad Hooters to her style ran the first foster home. She had, it turned out, twenty-five pit bulls. "They're all labs," she said.

A guy, who likely just dropped out of school or got out of prison, was mopping up the gross floor when we entered. He ushered us over to a rag-gedy stained couch, took away a flea-bitten child in diapers lurking among the pit bull pack, and left us with the pups. I whispered to Tim, "Do you see a Confederate flag?"

"No," he whispered back.

The dogs were old. Despite my insistence on a housebroken pooch—be-cause I have cancer, folks, and I'm useless to everyone after 4 p.m. and I need a copious amount of free time—I found myself wanting a baby.

Can I just get a puppy without emotional baggage?

No abandonment issues?!?

I just want a baby without any goddamn fear of abuse or starvation.

I have freakin' cancer, and I need my books, my writing, my pseudo-social life on social media (*I talk to no one*), my kids, and Tim. I'm frightfully dependent on him, in probably a psychotic way. And I want a puppy!

"We'll be touch," we lied, shuffling out of the crack house.

From there, we went to a park all the way in Mesa to meet a lady with a baby lab. I can respect the foster family's wishes to keep us out of their home.

There was Snickers.

A puppy. Without baggage.

Unlikely a lab.

I'll tell you how this will unfold. We'll keep Snickers. He'll stay. We are—this is a trait both Tim and I share to varying degrees—notoriously short-sighted with a high tolerance for pain. The puppy will work out. Already, I love him. So we'll muddle through this.

But stress.

The puppy stresses me out. He jumps nonstop, snaps, chews on shit, eats paper.

And I know about stress.

My stress is a hard ball, a tumor. So tight, so hard, a tiny fetal fist, knuckles that do not unravel, the fingers of a beast. My stress is alive, a death growing inside, cancer cells multiplying.

I believe this.

I believe I birthed my own cancer. It was born from my own stress, kept in my breast, fed like an evil garden in an enchanted and wicked forest on nutrients I unwillingly and willingly gave it.

The dog seems metaphoric. A good thing, eventually.

This dog is like my marriage.

I had an ultrasound and a CT scan recently. There was a small ache in my arm (which is now gone), and my doctor kindly catered to my paranoia. The ultrasound ruled out a blood clot.

Tomorrow is chemo. I just found out the results of my CT scan, and I'll see my oncologist tomorrow. This may be nothing, but there appears to be a nodule on my lung. It's too small to biopsy. *That* small. If it were lung cancer, it would be very early—Tim's specialty! It might've been there for a long, long time. It also looks like there are some cysts on my liver. Cysts. They don't look like cancer. I'll be having a PET Scan next.

I may be giving cancer more than one year.

26

Hire a Nanny! (December 2, 2015)

I showed Melody a photo of my bare breasts. Her sister still hasn't seen them. I asked her, "Are they weird?"

Melody looked at the photo and said, "No." She hesitated. "They're a little uneven."

Well, here we go. The nodule on my lung: Thirty to 40 percent of people who get CT scans will discover that they, too, have nodules. These are harmless. I may be one of those people. Or I may not. (*Probably not.*)

But it's very small, at .5 centimeters wide. Too small to biopsy—they like for them to be at least one centimeter before they dig in. We have to watch to see if it grows; I'll have another CT scan in six weeks. If it has grown, they'll dig in—small or not. But there's an unhappy risk: *puncturing a lung.*

Say it's cancerous, which they doubt. Then it's considered to be *metastasized breast cancer*—not some new cancer. That it is a separate, discrete cancer is statistically rare (*unless, of course, you're Jennifer Spiegel. Then, the sky's the limit . . .*).

Then, I would move from Stage Two Breast Cancer to Stage Four Breast Cancer.

Just like that!

There are also "cysts" on my liver, which the radiologists think are nothing at all, just cysts. But, well, I've had bad experiences with radiologists.

I'm having an MRI this upcoming week. If they're not cysts, they need to be removed—and their positioning is precarious.

Couldn't they move a little to the right, a little to the left?

That's the update: a CT scan in six weeks to check out the nodule on the lung and an MRI within the week to check on the cysts in the liver. Really, that's all I've got for you.

I told Tim, "If I die, you'll need a nanny."

Tim responded, "Even if you don't die, we should get a nanny." He paused. "She can watch TV with us . . . ."

My hair is coming back. It's white.

That's different.

27

And Now Back to Cancer!
(December 20, 2015)

I finished (again) my novel, which is about dying and sleeping. Or drugs and marriage. Or survival and bitterness. My novel is perpetually on the cusp of completion. I thought it was done in December 2014, again in April 2015, and then once more in December 2015. It's my best work to date, maybe, possibly, probably. Or not.

I finished grading English 101 compositions. It was an OK semester— not my best, but not my worst. (During my worst, I told a student, "Do us a favor: don't reproduce.") I told these students I had cancer.

Mostly, they were nice or they didn't care.

I wonder if they noticed I was wearing a wig. No one asked.

They ignored the hot flashes.

And . . . I finished chemo!

Sucked that poison right up through a port into my chest!

The chemo nurses in the chemo room give you cards and make a big deal about finishing treatment. I brought treats for everyone—like bringing in cookies for the class.

But I have to be honest: The *real* big deal for me was getting back the results of my CT and PET scans.

Chemo really wasn't that bad, except for the fact that I went bald, lost my eyebrows, lost my eyelashes, became annoyingly exhausted and increasingly antisocial and often irritable, never slept soundly, got strangely dried and cracked hands and feet, and was prematurely launched into menopause so I hot-flash anywhere from five to ten times a day (not to mention the nights, in

which I burrow into the quilts and then whip them off three minutes later).
Oh, and let's not talk marriage and sex and kids.

It wasn't that bad.

For such candor, I've said little about sex.

Tim and I almost had a good time (in chemo).

Except at the end, in which Tim grew weary of me (*I'm dying here, Tim*),
and I grew anxious over the scans (*I'm dying here, Tim*).

Once, he said, "You're playing the cancer card."

I was, like, "Um, yeah?"

(For the record, chemo wasn't that bad—but breast reconstruction *was
not fun*: insomnia, pain, Klonopin now nightly—I'm probably an addict and
will need to figure out how and when to wean myself off narcotics.)

But we had a good time: days off, lunch out, paper cups of coffee in our
hands. We'd arrive to chemo like rock stars. Tim, all buff. Me, glamourous red
wig on top of my head. Dark sunglasses, the both of us. Barely middle-aged.
Our drinks full and sloshing in sober merriment.

We were about to put on a show, and we knew it.

Many, many kind people (everyone was so nice) greeted us, and I'd toss
back my head but not too far back lest my wig slip, and I'd wave like the Queen
of England. We switched into high gear: Tim and I could be so funny for two
depressives.

I have no clue, now, in retrospect, how our comedy routine went; I just
know that we were loud and full of quips and observations and ease and grace-
less grace.

Someone would whisper to me, "You could be hired to perform at birthday parties."

(I'm not kidding.)

Someone else whispered, "You're so lucky to have someone like him go
through this with you." (She was not the first to say this.)

I thought about responding, "How do you think I ended up here? *This
man gave me the cancer.*"

I sometimes would. That's how our show might go.

We were on fire.

For, like, ten minutes.

Then, Tim would play Sudoku while I would happily read books and sip
my coffee.

What a great afternoon!

Following chemo, we went home to, as Tim put it, "an exquisite meal"
that one of my guardian angels—*that food signup sheet!*—had prepped for us,
a meal I'd never actually have the skills to make, with or without cancer.

A pretty good day!

But it had ended. And we had a stack of cards from the nurses.

You'll remember that we also got a dog and a bunch of scans were ordered for me due to mysterious cysts in my liver and a nodule on my lung.

Also, I'm not going to lie: *That puppy bites.*

And don't get mad at me for saying this: *He stinks, too.*

And: *Actually, he's just gross.*

I grew up with labs and retrievers. They're better.

I'm like, didn't I just carve out a little cancer time for myself in which I worked on two books at once, read excellent fiction nonstop, analyzed *The Walking Dead*, and still managed the wife/mom gig in a so-so fashion? *WTF?*

Ugh. Did I just write *WTF*? Next, I'll be using *LOL*. And *My bad.*

All of my efforts to get rid of Snickers have been thwarted.

Before that last chemo, prior to our big show, while we waited for the scan results in my oncologist's office, I said to Tim, "I'll tell you this: If the results of the scans reveal anything suspicious—*anything*—I'm getting rid of that dog."

Tim tried to "reason" with me. "Even if something were suspicious, you would still need a biopsy, which could take weeks. We don't need to get rid of the dog now."

I kinda lost it and said, "He goes *now*." And then I got mean. "It's me or the dog."

Tim got mad.

It was right then—Tim about to tell off his chemo-stricken, bald wife—that my oncologist whipped open the door and declared, "So, good news! Your scans don't reveal anything unusual!"

This is pretty much saying that I'm cancer-free (or, in all honesty, as close as I can ever get to saying I'm cancer-free).

I turned to Tim. "So I guess we're keeping the dog."

Tim, for his part, did put his arm around me.

I'll give him that.

The scan results alleviated about 70 percent of my stress. (There are technical terms for what they think the abnormalities are—and they will need to be watched.) I can't really say I'm happy about the dog.

If I'm "cancer-free," can I do that to my kids? Get rid of their puppy?

No. The dog stays.

But that was it. Chemo is over. Now, we're onto the next part. There's a second surgery, which we're scheduling soon, to remove the hard boob stuff and replace it with silicon bags. Shortly thereafter, radiation—which is killing me and saving me at the same time.

28

Tattoo Me (December 26, 2015)

Y es, I'm serious.

I really do plan on tattooing my faux-breasts in large, asymmetric, *are-you-kidding-me* tattoos.

The idea of completing my reconstruction with fake nipples (*nipple nipple nipple*) strikes me as, well, *absurd*: CRAZY—as if we're pretending that these unreal, falsified body parts are somehow OK. Tattoos, in contrast, are admissions, acceptances, and a claim. A claim on what, you ask?

I saw Facebook posts, wild tattoos over damaged bodies. When I saw them, I really knew that I needed to go in that direction.

I reposted a few shots of breasts with sprawling, striking art reclaiming losses.

Controversy launched!

(I edit now in May 2017. In retrospect, this was the beginning of the end, my fall from grace, when I gradually began to slink out of the favor of my very supportive cancer community, who were largely, but not exclusively, Christians. And I feel as if this is important to mull over. Sometimes, I would imagine that it was my incessant cussing, but it was *this*: My breast exposure, my revelry, my worldliness. Tattoo-pangs would be followed by vigilant anti-Trump politics which I will edit out of this book because it's not a book on politics and I seriously went ballistic. Politics, though, had a strange effect on my cancer life. Gradually, I became "well." Gradually, my faithful supporters— so truly wonderful—became disenchanted with this real Jennifer, this Jennifer craving raucous tattoos, this Jennifer of the unflinching politics. Hence, right here, we are at the beginning of the end, a crossroads. And could I not have waited? Could I have kept some things secret? For the sake of their fidelity? Their loving care? Must I speak of breasts—bare, stained, patterned? Shouldn't I have kept the national political landscape away from my heart, dismissing it as worldly when I am not of this world? Hadn't I stepped too far outside of my stricken box?)

I got emails from offended friends after I posted naked, tattooed breasts. I was surprised.

So, let me tell you about these breasts underneath these tattoos painted over mastectomies and reconstructions . . . .

First, the woman had a disease that might kill her. *Kill her.*

Second, the disease was extensive enough to warrant complete removal of the breast, rather than a lumpectomy. Perhaps there was chemo; we don't know. The nipple, too, had to go.

Third, a tissue expander was stitched into her body, and a big scar bisected her chest—where the breast once was.

Fourth, she went in weekly to expand the tissue, which means she went in to have her old skin stretched in ways that really are miraculous, painful, and *unnatural*. This was done by injecting a needle right where her missing nipple used to be and filling the expander, incrementally, with gunk. (I'm still not entirely sure what that gunk is—liquid silicon?)

Fifth, she was in pain after each "fill," and sleeping was difficult because she had to sleep on her back or her side, ever conscious of her *very hard* fake breasts (*hard* like a doll's head).

Sixth, she finally stopped the fills when she felt like she *looked*—not *felt*—normal enough.

Seventh, she had a second surgery in which the scar was reopened, the tissue expanders were removed, and a soft implant was put inside. Now, all she wanted was to sleep and not have strange armor sewn into her body.

Eighth, she finally had a fake breast that looked fine with clothes on. It wasn't her, of course. There was no sensation—or, if there were, it was minimal. The scar remained. She was, pretty much, disassociated from the falsity, but thankful for its presence nonetheless. She could go out in public.

Ninth, after one full year (it's best to wait a year), she decided to tattoo the faux breast, transforming that which was diseased into—quite simply, quite perfectly—*art*. This is the claim.

At least, it's my claim.

Breasts have power. I'm not really prepared to philosophize on breasts, but the obvious issue is how closely they are tied to identity, to womanhood. To remove them is to call into question identity and womanhood. A woman may deal with this in a number of ways. She may have confidence in her own person, her own feminism. She may not have that confidence. She may feel the onslaught of the breast cancer, which has now—she's sure—left her desexualized, asexualized: a nonsexual being.

Actually, just *ugly*.

I have thought this: *Is reconstruction a cop-out?*

Is reconstruction an admission that I lack the confidence to deal with the loss of the symbolic value of a breast?

Am I admitting that I need that *crutch*—which, in this case, is a fake boob?

Am I making a lame stab at normalcy (*looking normal*, that is—not feeling normal, which is not on my list of expectations)?

Is that what reconstruction is all about?

Is there some inner strength that I do not possess involved in the decision to remain flat-chested?

I don't have answers to those questions.

Is a photo of a reconstructed breast, tattooed, pornographic?

No.

It is an aesthetic claim. It is to make art of oneself, to take one's loss and turn it into something beautiful. To confuse this with porn or something base is to misunderstand art, which is about beauty, goodness, and truth. There is a distinction between art and porn, and nudity is not *intrinsically* pornographic.

Michelangelo's *David*?

I think the important thing in this discussion, then, really doesn't have as much to do with tattoos as it does with the distinction between art and pornography. If that distinction is clear, the tattooed, reconstructed breast is anything but offensive.

P.S.—I'm anti-porn.

That kind of comment gets me in trouble. I'm suddenly moralistic! Simply put, I think porn is dehumanizing to men and women, distorts the goodness of human sexuality, and objectifies women (mostly). Porn is gross.

This objectification is the thing here. Allow me to go all biblical. Remember the whole Adam-in-the-Garden-of-Eden saga? One of his God-given tasks was to *name the animals*. Give them names. The implication is that names are unique, fitting, particular, chosen with purpose. If you've named your baby, you know how it goes. You want the name to be special.

Names are important, then. We use Jane Doe or John Doe to designate everywoman and everyman. We are impressed or touched or attentive when we are addressed by our names. In terms of race, we know there's a dishonorable, dehumanizing thing happening when a black man is referred to as "boy," rather than by his name. I could go on and on about this.

Adam didn't just call the animals anything. His naming project, in a sense, was the *opposite* of objectification. It required not just attention but giving the object an identity!

Tattoos are like names.

Women who are tattooing their reconstructed breasts are trying to re-associate what has been disassociated.

They are making claims on the territory of their skin.

They are rejecting the pornographic by insisting on an aesthetic identity.

Basically, they don't want that body part to be any breast; rather, they want it to be *their breast*.

Should this image be viewed?

Yes, of course.

Unless the breast is to be objectified.

29

Cancer, You've Had Over Six Months (January 1, 2016)

Happy New Year!

I don't want to be cynical and weird, a big downer on the first day of 2016.

In my fledgling literary career, I've been a big proponent of the redemptive end. So let's focus on this: *I'm all about the redemptive end.*

The redemptive end is not always a happy ending. It's just a meaningful ending. (My favorite example of the unhappy-but-redemptive ending might be *The Great Gatsby*.) An appropriate ending. An ending with *umph*, resolution, and truth. Yes, there is ultimate triumph in the narrative, even this very cancer narrative—but it may be triumph without me (our current protagonist).

So, goodbye to 2015!

What was your redemptive end?

Chemo concluded on December 16, 2015, and surgery is planned for January 13, 2016, to put in soft implants! (That's Tim's birthday, by the way, and I was just thinking that I sure hope I don't go into cardiac arrest on the operating table and *die*, because that might ruin the day for him.) I also got a new wig, which now looks silly to me.

Basically, though, I've been waiting to feel better. Supposedly, two weeks after chemo, one's bloodwork normalizes—which is required for the second breast surgery. I've been waiting.

It's not happening. I still feel weak, tired, irritable, et al.

I'm preoccupied with a few things at the beginning of this new year.

* * *

I have doubts about recovering. I know that the hair grows back, the eyebrows, the eyelashes. I wonder if I'll regain my strength, if I'll be able to function energetically after 6 p.m. Will I go out at night again? Will I leave the house after dark without Tim, my caretaker? Will I be able to tolerate my children's *childishness*? Will they grow up with a "sickly" mom?

I've always had this dread of those who suffer from some chronic weakness. I think it shows up in my unpublished novel: my dread, my fright, my anxiety—surrounding weakness.

And now I'm weak.

I've written about this already here. How we have these sickly types around us? There's usually one in our family. They've always got something. They can't come to the big event because they're tired or constipated or vomiting or they have this debilitating headache—and our kids are perpetually disappointed by their no-shows but used to them, too, and we accept it in ways that range from pandering and patronizing to empathy and compensation.

You know these people, don't you?

They fuck up our plans.

I've been intolerant.

I've lacked empathy.

I've loathed—in my heart of hearts—their inability to "fake it," to get up and carry the fuck on.

(My mother did it when my dad died in a car accident in 2002: *carried the fuck on.* That's the kind of women we are, the kind of woman I'm supposed to be.)

But now . . . .

I'm the sickly person, unable to carry-the-fuck-on.

And it scares me.

Is this my future? Tim is not inexperienced in dealing with the ill, sadly. Will this be our new dynamic? He will be there to care for me and give the kids a good time, a sense of normalcy?

Poor perpetually messed-up Tim will be their normalcy?

I will be the one who's too tired to go to the park, to play the game, to do anything?

This has been on my mind a lot.

* * *

I'm worried about my marriage. Oh, we'll stay married. Don't worry. But I'm stressed about the dynamic, the caretaker shift, the loss of equality. Being your spouse's ward is not sexy. I wonder if my marriage is *irreparably* different.

Interestingly, too, we've lost a bit of our comic relief—without our trips to chemo, where we would put on our weekly comedy shows.

* * *

I'm worried about this new state of the anxiety. Aches and pains are normal, yes? But now: an arm thing is bone cancer, a mark is skin cancer, my weariness is forever.

Sickly types talk symptoms, and now I talk symptoms.

So, 2016: *I wait for recovery.*

One of my friends told me she wished renewed hope in 2016 for me. That is the kindest wish.

Did I miss my redemptive end?

30

Going Secular (January 12, 2016)

An old college friend emailed me after reading some of my stuff and he said, "You sound more secular than you did a year ago."

Do I?

There's no need for surprise here. *Friend, I'm still the same Bible-thumper I was that day I accidentally fell into your arms at the ice-cream social in the dorm lobby that first week of our freshman year at the U. of A.*

(The Friend: West Ellis, who ran a bar—like, a real bar with hard liquor—from his dorm room in the honors dorm in college, who joined the Peace Corps upon graduation and went to Bolivia, who got married and had a kid and became a high school film and economics teacher on an Arizona Navajo reservation for years—a reservation bigger than the state of West Virginia—who sent me a Tig Notaro CD when I got cancer, who wrote me faithfully, who moved—weirdly—to Memphis, Tennessee, with his family. That West Ellis, haunting my life like a wraith, an angel.)

West, I'm just older now, less reserved or guarded or interested in pretense than I previously was—so my means of expressing my religious self are possibly more nuanced and complex, but more likely to offend?

What if what he calls *secular* I just call *candor*?

I still—*here it is, friend*—interpret my cancer entirely through the lens of religion.

I might need to address Christianity for the sake of narrative integrity, though, since this is a book about writing.

(One in eight women authors will get breast cancer.)

Why do I need to address religious belief in my non-informative guide to breast cancer? How do you *not*? I'm possibly dying here—*as are you*, but mine is more acutely possible—so there's nothing like a death threat, a real one, to crash your back against the wall and make you think about the meaning of life.

For me to avoid religion would be a cop-out.

My heathen friends shouldn't be alarmed. I have no intention of proselytizing, which is something I vigorously flee from, and one reason why I choose to write, mostly, for a secular audience. (About six or seven devoted Christians still read my stuff.)

I write for heathens!

As far as I'm concerned, my subject matter is Truth. Let's get lofty. To quote Picasso, "Art is a lie which makes us realize the truth." That's the epigraph to Chaim Potok's novel, *My Name Is Asher Lev*. (Please read this book as soon as possible.)

Hence, a cancer book on writing, a writing book on God: *the myth of secularity!*

I deliberately made a choice when I was youngish to write for secular audiences.

I did so primarily because I didn't want to be associated with a poor artistic aesthetic—and I tend to find Christian fiction or Christian literature or, even more generally speaking, Christian art stuff, not so hot, often second rate, imitative, unoriginal, sappy, simplistic. Thomas Kinkade sent me into melt-down mode.

I pretty much ran over to the other camp early on because that's where the real artists were. I knocked on the door and shouted, "Let me in! Let me in!" That's where F. Scott Fitzgerald and Ernest Hemingway and Lorrie Moore and Philip Roth wrote.

There are also amazing Christians doing art stuff in the secular world. Johnny Cash did it! Bono! James McBride! And . . . MY HEROINE . . . Marilynne Robinson (who would probably find me over the top)!

(Wait. Let's talk more about Marilynne Robinson. I don't know how a Calvinist woman from Idaho manages to write the most amazing works of fiction, winning every literary award, and getting to have intellectual conversations with the President of the United States and Jon Stewart—but she has. I admire her hugely, and though I write nothing like her whatsoever, I have to refer to her when I discuss my writing and my religion.)

* * *

Here's a story. *Let me tell you a story about the calling . . . .*

This is a book about writing, right?

When I was fourteen, I fell in love. With a shark. In Florida. The humidity left us wet and shiny, but we were young and beautiful. Or at least he was. He was nineteen. Not a shark at all, but his profile was sleek, smooth, like he could slice through the surface of things. He could glide through deep waters.

We were at a summer church retreat. I don't know why these revelers, these Holy Rollers, chose Florida for their speaking in tongues. Drenched, sweaty, tropical praise. Charismatic Baptists from around the world glowed, foreheads wet and glistening—hopeful that, one day, all the darkness in the world would be washed away. By love.

Pure and holy love.

Seeing this nineteen-year-old boy, I, girl-woman, thought I knew something about love. I didn't have to wait for the Rapture. Surely, this new, not-quite-sexual-but-rather-erotic wave of emotion for Shark bordered on the rapturous.

It seemed holy.

I was only a child: *Had I discovered God?*

The retreat was less than ten days long. Not much happened. Shark-sightings and ping-pong and cafeteria food and square-dancing intermingled with praise and prayer. Shark and I, despite my emerging womanliness, said nothing to one another—since, in reality, normal nineteen-year-olds aren't terribly interested in fourteen-year-olds.

At least, they weren't back then.

Much ado about nothing.

Nada.

The Big Nada, à la Hemingway.

I went home. To mourn. I embraced my persona. But there I was, a teen-ager newly defined by this: *my loss.*

I discovered Dostoyevsky, Duran Duran.

Duran Duran!

The loss of Shark seemed somehow monumental in defining who I was.

For at least a year, I kept a picture of a Great White pinned to my high school cubicle—so I could be clearly identified as one enslaved not by love, but by *unrequited love*—its deceptive and evil twin.

Did I mention the kicker?

Shark was Irish, from some small town in Northern Ireland. We were Protestants, so in the years that followed, I could engage in fantasies in which he died in revolution, in battle with the IRA. I could picture him in blue jeans and a white tee, barefoot, walking among concrete rubble from bombed-out buildings or through broken Irish glass (stained-glass windows belonging to churches) shadowed by ruins, a U2 song playing in the background. I could tear up appropriately during "Sunday Bloody Sunday."

The only other crazy thing about that summer was that I unexpectedly got my period and bled all over my Aunt Debbie's sheets when I went to Denver. The sole reason why this is worth mentioning is that, ironically, I got my period for the first time ever the previous summer. Guess where I was. You got it. *Aunt Debbie's in Denver.*

Bled all over her sheets two summers in a row!

Irony. Iron. Blood.

The end.

Most of this is true, but some of it isn't. This didn't take place in Florida. It wasn't a Baptist Charismatic thing. We were Presbyterians. In Minnesota.

I was never very charismatic.

Shark is real. We never had any interaction, but I did do a half-hearted search on the web once. That dug up something: he might be—I'm not entirely sure—a member of the *clergy* (!) in Northern Ireland.

A man o' God!

And the bleeding-at-Aunt-Debbie's stuff is real.

I did do something rather critical, in my little world, however: *I wrote it all down.* Turned it into a story.

I worked on that baby, too. I came home from school and wrote like a fiend. Before I turned fifteen, my shark incident had morphed into fiction.

This was the calling.

The manuscript no longer exists, and there are no traces that it once did. *Thank God.* Because it SUCKED!

S S S S S S U U U U U U U U U C C C C C C C C K - KKKKKKKKEEEEEEEDDDDDDD!!!!!

Oh, it was bad.

Handwritten, I think.

It pains me to think about how bad it was.

But I have no problem telling you the details of my delusional romance or first menstrual cycle. Why was this event so significant?

The inherent lessons: Shark, for that's how he became known to me, transformed from fact to fiction, from particular to universal, from a cute boy to an objective correlative. In these transformations, I learned about story. I learned that a story can resonate and resonate and resonate.

I learned that my loss might be your solace.

Story can get at truth. It can get at universals. It's magical.

A story can inform you in non-informative ways.

I can write a non-informative guide.

* * *

If I were writing this Shark story now, I'd play with romantic love and the Rapture. I'd use the period thing, turn it into metaphor. The cliché about how it marks the beginning of womanhood. I could use that. I didn't deliberately christen Shark with the name of a predator, but that's good. I think he was a nice guy, so that Shark moniker might be perceived as unkind. But, hey, fiction involves the manipulation of details—in service of the universal.

And there is the longing, the desire, the taint and smudge of eroticism, the emptiness.

So my summer of shark-sightings was a personal and professional season. I suppose I could write how I mistook a boy for God, and how this impacted my life for, like, decades. Boys for gods! Professionally, I tasted the sweetness of writing. When Shark disappeared, writing did not.

Will I say the same about cancer?

Might a story about cancer morph into writing truisms?

And so, here's my official statement on the perceived secularization. My allegiance is to Truth, and good art is about Truth, even when it's fiction.

Is that secular, West?

* * *

David Bowie died of cancer on Sunday. He made Art of himself. He embodied an aesthetic, using himself as a palette. Rest in peace, David.

31

Is This Part II? (January 17, 2016)

Ah, well, here we are.

Looking for that Redemptive End!

My breasts are now soft, more or less "done." When we took off the bandage, which Tim unraveled in mock-seduction, harking back to either mummification or women in history who bound their breasts, I did feel relief, a tinge of *I'm done.*

Of course I'm not. Radiation is next.

Still: I felt it. *The Grand Return of Soft Boobies!* How miraculous is it that doctors can make breasts?

I've been flirting with the idea of going without the wig, showing up with the subtle sheen of silver peached over my scalp. I've considered it, now that I'm less Melissa Etheridge and more Annie Lennox.

The port is gone too. He removed it during surgery.

While I no longer can crack open nuts on my bare chest, I seem to regularly emit a strange squishy sound. You know the sound: *glub, glub?* There's this *glub, glub* sound coming from inside my body.

Ah, now, here we are.

I'm still thinking about the act of writing. About this memoir: Apart from the journalistic detail any "survivor" with implants could tell you, what will this narrative reveal?

I really want to write the cancer book that hasn't been written.

What is *The Untold Breast Cancer Story?*

So maybe it's about writing. And maybe it's about God.

And maybe it's about my marriage.

119

Maybe.

* * *

That image: the unraveling of bandaged breasts. Did he pull the ribbon from one stationary spot? Did I spin slowly? Did I dance like Salome? Did we stand before a mirror? What happened in that moment, our attention fixed on flesh?

Can you picture the unraveling, a bride on her wedding night?

There are other untold breast cancer stories. But mine might reside here. We are standing there, post-surgery, cancer-weary, Annie-Lennoxed, marriage-enmeshed, caught up in it, wondering when or if a sweet life resumes/ gets started. The *Now what?* of life hitting home with my new breasts, both touchable and untouchable. *Where to?*, we might ask, now that we're swabbing lotion on and removing cotton from our wounds.

Is this Part II?

First, we were one kind of person; now, we are another.

The softness of my spiritual skin, the underbelly of my religiosity, exposed.

My body, dissected, shorn, rebuilt, unreal.

I look at Tim now, post cancer. I thought I knew him well.

And now I know him better.

32

Divorce (undated)

I've been thinking about severance: separation, partition, uncoupling. Breasts from body, husbands from wives, mothers from kids, friend from friend. Not just loss, but detachment.

I begin radiation—the thing that kills you to save you—on February 15, President's Day. There will be six weeks of it. Yesterday, I got four teeny, tiny tattoos—dots to mark me under the beam, so that the radiation hits the same spot every time. Smaller, really, than freckles. I met with the radiation oncologist on Wednesday. We discussed my breasts, the statistics surrounding my life or death, lymphedema caused by scratches and wounds and dog bites. (We hit it off, this guy and I: "*You've* got a puppy? *I've* got a puppy!" We pulled out our phones, searching for photos. "Here's *my* puppy! And here's *my* puppy!" My fake breasts, silicon puffed, ready for his clinical scrutiny. But breasts aside: "Look at my puppy! Just look at my pup!")

My hair is curiously *chic*. Annie Lenox, silver. I'm anxious to try it out in public, this other me, this not-at-all me, this vogue girl with the buzz cut. I don't think Tim is gung-ho. Tim likes his women girly. I knew this from the beginning, never quite fulfilling the role (*not fulfilling it at all*). I acquiesced by keeping my hair longer than I would have. But, as I'm searching his face for secret knowledge, I'm seeing hesitation. He's all, *If you want to try it, try it*. But I'm seeing, *Are you really wanting to look so mannish?* Which is a nice way of saying *butch*. Which is really saying *not feminine*. He's always hated my mind-reading tactics, which he says are often/usually wrong—but you know are *totally right*.

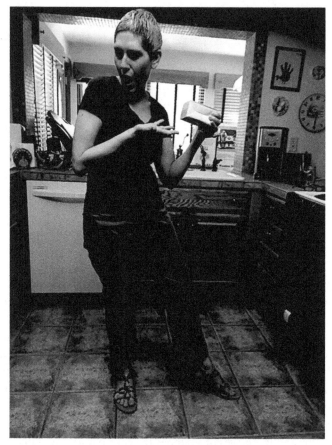

Photo by Melody Bell.

The hot flashes persist. Actually, they *rage*. Rage, rage. With a new addition: cold flashes. I think they're new? I don't remember. While at one point I'm dripping sweat and stripping off clothes, at another time I'm bone-chillingly cold—*inconsolably* cold. Whatever it is that will warm me is surely something from within. The blankets do not help. Layers and layers of false comforters.

Then, my fingernails are yellowed, uneven moons of stained or stripped gold, rust. They look thick, fungal.

Also, Tim and I have been talking a lot about sex. To be vague, we've discussed *how, why, when*—but not really *where, who,* or *what*.

I thought maybe I should discuss this with a doctor—have you discussed sex with a doctor before?

Everyone gets all pseudo-professional and faux-clinical, but there's the stench of fraud in the air.

I'm not sure with which doctor to discuss it.

My plastic surgeon, who I vowed not to speak unkindly about as we have mutual friends (weird!) and he's the bastion of professional expertise, doesn't seem like the type in which to confide.

The medical oncologist, my personal favorite, would probably blush. A sweet, kind man, of East Indian descent.

The radiation oncologist looks like he could handle it. After all, we got personal and discussed our puppies. But he's sorta like a buddy.

I asked one of my friends who had cancer about sex, and she said something like, "You'll know when the time is right."

Are you serious?

The time is never right!

Finally, also, I think I've picked my tattoo artist. I've never seen his work.

He was born in East Germany and smuggled over the Berlin War during the Cold War. He was then adopted by Americans and raised here in the United States. Now a tattoo artist, he's a former sniper in the U.S. Army.

Escaped orphan-turned-sniper. *He's the one.*

Why? For the story of it. Turn my body into Art, into story.

Do it, Sniper.

May I call you "Sniper"?

Swiper, no swiping.

I choose him for his metaphoric value: his own separation story, separated from his family, adopted by another, having crossed over a partition that divided West from East by a monolithic, dystopian, Orwellian Great Wall. I want for his ink to stain my skin, to absorb that story into my own.

Separation, partition, uncoupling, and detachment. I am detached from my body. I can talk pets with the same doctor who will blast me with radiation, make me nuclear. I can talk to him while wearing a paper dress, open in the front, body exposed.

I am utterly disconnected from my body.

Funny, but I'm not disconnected from the hair. That hair is too personal, too much of me. Saying, *You're not really chic, bitch.* Saying, *You don't look like a girl to me.*

Where is my ability to disassociate?

Hot flashes, cold flashes, fingernails: a body at war. The East and West Berlin of my body.

And sex, oh sex, the great enemy.

Cancer is a lonely endeavor, a hot and cold place, brittle in parts, soft in others, dotted to designate borders, a no man's land over my heart.

33

Dear Wendy and Melody, Part I
(February 14, 2016)

Dear Wendy and Melody,

You're growing up on me! I should've been more prepared for this. Here I was, thinking how I'd write you letters telling you all kinds of motherly wisdom, and I'd tell you how special you each are, and how much I love both of you—but then this "tween" bullshit started happening, circumventing my plans.

I noticed the music right away. It's Melody more than Wendy, but it's happening: this interest in pop music. I hear names. I hear Taylor Swift mentioned. Katy Perry. Adele, if I'm lucky. I'm apprehensive. I don't think Daddy is, but he's always been the fun one. I know how this goes. I've been there. I remember.

Actually, it's different now.

When I was a child, I was immediately launched into desire for men. I don't think it was sexual—I really don't—but I remember feeling something I'd call love for Shawn Cassidy! And then Tom Selleck. And shortly thereafter, or maybe simultaneously, Rick Springfield, who I *really* loved. And, of course, Duran Duran, where my love got mixed up with a trashy understanding of art. I loved many, many men. Beautiful men who told me what they liked in a woman. I was your age or younger when I started seeing myself through the eyes of men. I don't even remember the women, until maybe Madonna. But those men taught me things.

Last night, Daddy and I failed to go out on our first date since cancer. So, of course, like a girl properly trained in the ways of objectification, I reasoned that we didn't go out because I'm ugly, I'm not sexy, I'm not woman enough for your father.

And now, I see you, my own babies, my pretty girls, in the initial throes of a kind of androgynous lust. Their gaze is on other girls, I think. Other girls are showing them what it means to be a woman.

As a mom, I think about my options. I've seen moms censor everything; I've seen moms permit anything. I remember my own lost years—*years*—enslaved, enslaved to an impossible romantic ideal. I see myself now, still visibly estranged from the feminine, and I want for you to avoid this kind of suffering, this heartbreak.

You will learn things. I'm not going to stop you. I'm not going to forbid rock n' roll. I will not force you to analyze lyrics. I will not make you feel guilty for singing those inane songs.

I don't buy the argument that this is just a part of growing up, though.

I don't think you need to necessarily fall into some kind of pop music/romantic fool trap. But I'm feeling a little disillusioned: banning the crap music, pulling the plug on the dance music, getting weird every time a teeny-bopper struts her sexualized stuff seems outlandish to me.

Will you—I didn't want for this happen—become like me?

Daddy and I didn't go on our date. I guess all those weekly trips to chemo can count as dates. I'm sure we spent more time alone together this year than any other married couple I know, and I'm not saying this facetiously.

We watched a movie with you two, a stupid movie, and I hate to say it, but your dad just doesn't get it.

In this movie—which we can just call *Dumbass Movie Geared Towards Prepubescent Girls*—there was the obvious stuff: the teenagers and their looks and their ways and their songs and all that crap. Then, there was the introduction of romance, which will now be the prevailing theme of almost every single movie, TV show, and book you will encounter for the rest of your lives.

I just want to tell you this: *It's coming at you, and it's not going to stop.*

Yesterday, in *Dumbass Movie Geared Towards Prepubescent Girls*, the prince said to the girl (I'm paraphrasing), "Tell me one thing about yourself that no one else knows."

It's very unlikely that a guy will ever say this to you.

Yesterday, in *Dumbass Movie Geared Towards Prepubescent Girls*, the prince said to the girl (I'm paraphrasing), "I've said enough. I want to hear from you."

It's also very unlikely that a guy will ever say this to you.

Yesterday, in *Dumbass Movie Geared Towards Prepubescent Girls*, the prince said to the girl (I'm paraphrasing), "I'll teach you."

This, he might say.

He might want to teach you noble things, but he also might be gently, sweetly, falsely trying to teach you ignoble things.

Your response may surprise you. You may try your hardest to be somehow adorable, witty, engaging, and smart in an effort to get him to talk about himself some more. You may reveal very little about yourself, actually—but it's unlikely that he'll notice.

Your turn to talk will quickly be up! He'll start again!

I'm sorry I'm so cynical, girls. I got scared during *Dumbass Movie Geared Towards Prepubescent Girls.* I saw what's ahead.

And what if I'm not here to help you? What if you don't have a mom to talk to?

Girls, can you weather the storm coming?

Will you find your voices?

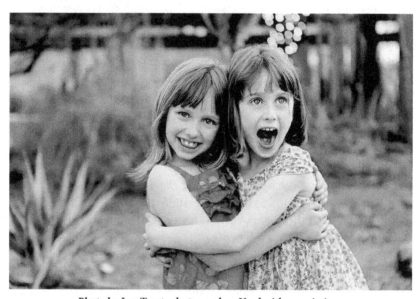

Photo by Lex Treat, photographer. Used with permission.

34

Cancer Was My Writing Sabbatical (February 2016)

"Cancer was my writing sabbatical." I said this to my friend the other day, as if I were joking.

I wasn't.

Siobhan responded, "It would be a good title for your memoir."

I like *Where the Fuck Is Tim?* Better.

Memoir, as a topic, has weighed heavily on me as I started "treatment" (they keep referring to radiation as my *treatment*, which is a word I like as much as I like *survivor* in this cancer context). Is it supposed to sound like a facial?

For *treatment*, they open my paper gown to line up my tiny tattoos with a machine that hovers or roves (yes, it *roves*) over me like some kind of space-age hibernation tank (think Sigourney Weaver in *Alien*), zapping me invisibly, in a deceptively simple way. Radiation is simple.

There is only a green light and a prolonged buzz.

The prolonged buzz is the sole cue that I'm in danger.

* * *

And it happened.

I was heading to radiation, now daily at 8:30 a.m. I had to drop the kids off at school along the way, and I just didn't want to put the wig on.

I left the house without it.

I'll never put it back on.

* * *

Going to my girls' school has been tough. I know people there. My girls are embarrassed by my hair. Kids stare. That's what children do. They do not know how to kindly look away.

Melody is especially embarrassed. Her little friends ogle, unabashedly. So this is what it must be like. *God help the disabled, the burn victims.* Melody tries to act as if it's no big deal. But it's tough for her. She's eight. Her mom is almost bald. And yet I'm hurt by her embarrassment.

I think, also, about how she doesn't want to take this one water bottle to school with my oncologist's logo on it. We have to put it in a sock, hiding the logo: She's embarrassed by my cancer.

And then I remember how Tim was on her "side." He didn't try to talk her out of her embarrassment. He didn't say, "Your mother's cancer is nothing to be ashamed about."

She was allowed to be embarrassed over her mother's deadly disease.

I showed up at the vet's without my wig, too. I've known my vet for some twenty years. Once, I saw him with his wife at a Dave Matthews concert. On another time, my family ran into his family at a California Pizza Kitchen.

He was the first one *ever* who asked about my hair. "What's this?"

"No one ever asks," I said. "They just stare or pretend not to notice."

Later, I told Tim.

Tim said, "Did he tell you it looked nice?"

"No. That wouldn't be right. You don't say that to a married woman."

"Sure you do," he said. "Well, what did he say?"

"We talked about cancer." I paused. "And then the dog."

* * *

My creative writing students are the best. Cancer is a story, my body a narrative, hair a flourish, an accent. They just move along.

* * *

For Tim, it's all the same, which is to say he's immune, which is to say he's indifferent. Cancer is no narrative; it's a scourge.

* * *

He isn't in this with me like he was with chemo. It doesn't make sense for him to go to radiation with me every day for ten minutes. So he's removed from the complications of this cancer moment. The *treatments*, the hair.

I am alone in my hibernation tank.

* * *

One of my new breasts is definitely smaller than the other. After only three days of radiation, I noticed.

I was warned: radiation can cause tissue-damage, hardening. Shrinking, shriveling, disfigurement.

After only three zaps?

But it's obvious.

So now: a new situation. I spent over five months with tissue expanders sewn into my body. They're finally soft. Not terribly huge. My intention is still to tattoo them wildly. Will I put asymmetrical, tattooed breasts on the cover of my book?

My boobs on the cover. That has always been my intention.

My intention has been to remove buffers, to scorn self-protection, to reveal my bare breasts.

Can I turn my breasts into universals?

What is a memoir, after all, if not a life rendered universal?

Can't I make something of this cancer?

* * *

I spent three hours at the Urgent Care with Wendy on Sunday night. I pretty much knew she had strep, so I wasn't fraught with fear.

We had spent the previous day, Saturday, at the Renaissance Festival, celebrating Wendy's tenth birthday—with a bunch of her friends.

But it wasn't the party that I had wanted.

I had wanted to, somehow, thank all the moms who watched my kids and drove them places while I had chemo. I imagined an elaborate scenario in which I'd give their kids this fabulous time, a rollicking/jovial/historically relevant good time—while simultaneously celebrating the birth of my own daughter. I nobly footed the bill for all tickets.

And that's where my nobility ended.

It was, like, the hottest day of the year so far.

I had five million kids and a handful of kindly adults in a crowd of a billion freaks and carnies dressed in this whacky fusion between Steampunk Renaissance garb and Shakespearean costume that accentuated the bosom. And there is no other word to use besides *bosom*. We are not talking about *breasts*. These were *bosoms*. Lots and lots of *bosoms*.

On the pretense of saying *thank you*, I had adults drive out into the middle of nowhere in the Arizona desert. Two kids had to take Dramamine. One kid threw up. However, on the way home, in our car, appropriately medicated, the puker did an amazing rendition of "Let It Go." *At the top of her lungs.*

Tim joined her, turning to me in shotgun and singing, "The cold never bothered me anyway."

On the pretense of saying *thank you*, I paid for their tickets . . . .

And then the adults were forced to buy chicken skewered on sticks, bottled water on demand, turkey legs, hot pretzels, and—in some cases—garlands of flowers to wear on the heads of young Renaissance virgins. The adults were forced to escort kids to toilets, apply sunscreen, give up their hats to children who forgot theirs, book it across the festival to get to the sword-swallowing show or the jousting tournament or the acrobats who told bawdy sex jokes.

On the pretense of saying *thank you*, I gathered people together—and *worked* their asses.

They kept *me* shaded, gave *me* water, and took care of each other.

Then, to top it all off, strep spread throughout the party.

On the pretense of saying *thank you*, I sent all their kids home sick.

One is hospitalized now.

I wish I were joking.

Tim said, "All part of the thank-you package."

So, Wendy ended up in Urgent Care on Sunday night. I played the cancer card when we got there, hoping they'd see us more quickly. I told the receptionist, "I actually have cancer—would you tell a doctor?—and I probably shouldn't be in the waiting room with sick people?"

The Urgent Care staff nodded, and escorted Wendy and me into our own room—where we waited for three hours to see the doctor.

Boom.

Wendy, who's a cute kid, looked horrible—red eyes, watery, messed up. She leaned on me for half the time. She tried to sleep on my leg for a bit, leaving drool.

I told myself that this is a privilege. It is the privilege of being alive. This is why I wanted to live: *so my kids would grow up with a mother on whose leg they could drool while sitting with them in the Urgent Care.*

She was, indeed, diagnosed with strep.

35

Dear Wendy and Melody, Part II

Inspired by Nora Ephron (undated)

In an essay called "What I Wish I'd Known," Nora Ephron wrote, "There's no point in making pie crust from scratch." She realized this as an adult. It's not worth it.

I'd like to tell my daughters twenty-five things right now (in case, I can't be there)—some serious, some not so serious. And I have other things to say to them, too; this is not comprehensive at all. I'd be so bummed if this were considered the whole of my motherly message to Wendy and Melody, Woo and Moo.

But here we go:

- Don't argue with each other over stupid stuff.

- Don't flip out over a couple bad grades. Wendy, this one is for you. If you get a "B" or even a "C," who cares?

- Even if you don't like the President of the United States, I think you should speak respectfully about him or her. [Note from the future: I ended up violating this one hugely when Trump was elected, so—not to justify myself—but maybe there is philosophical justification for opposition.]

- Read all the time. Try to read a book a week. Fiction, nonfiction, classics, contemporary stuff. If you want to read garbage, it's OK—but read mostly the good stuff, and do it voraciously. Melody, you can read at a higher level than you think you can. I totally know this is true.

- If you ask me, and you haven't, I'd be super diligent in studying the arts and history. I'm sure your dad would mention science. Which is to say, then, be learners, listeners, students, readers.

- Be a little weirded out by people who don't like animals. What's up with that?

- Daddy's probably right about being fun and adventurous, but I'm right about washing your hands often.

- Be adamantly against racism.

- Since this is a secular memoir (written for heathens and five or six Christians), I'll keep it simple: Try to keep the Ten Commandments.

- You are girls. There's so much to say here, but please make sure you can take care of yourselves. You may need to watch TV alone, like Grandma. You might need to be a single mom. Things happen in life, and being a woman alone is not always easy. There is more to being a woman than what I am saying here, but be able to take care of yourself financially.

- Don't let men fuck with you. I mean it. *Do. Not. Let. Men. Fuck. With. You.*

- Which reminds me: There are no bad words. There are contexts in which it is inappropriate for you to use certain words. This is another reason why you should read a lot. If you find yourself in a situation where a real zinger might be appropriate, you'll be able to quote Mark Twain or Dorothy Parker rather than drop an F-bomb.

- I'd personally recommend not coloring your hair. It's a trap.

- Don't be snobby or too vicious like me; don't be too moody like your dad.

- Don't marry a guy who doesn't make you laugh. Is this all I have to say on this topic? *It is not.*

- Try to travel.

- Don't do drugs. Why bother with that shit?

- Melody, eat your freakin' vegetables.

- Wendy, would you drink more water, girlfriend?

- Melody, you might be one of the popular girls. I'm sensing it now. Don't ever be mean to the unpopular girls. *Ever.* And this popular thing: It's OK, but be voracious in your search for goodness, for beauty, for truth— which might be in unpopular realms.

- Wendy, you're a bit of a perfectionist. You can tone it down. It's OK if your handwriting is a little messy. It's even OK if you get a color-change at school. If you mess up, don't fall apart. It's fine. That combination of perfectionism and fragility is not so hot.

- Grandma's nuts, but you can rely on her.

- Hold on tightly to the good people in your life.

- Be one of those people interested in the meaning of life.

- If you've agreed to do something for someone or be somewhere, do what you said you'd do. Do not be a flake.

36

Anxiety Attack (March 9, 2016)

I've been filled with anxiety.

* * *

Tim's allergies.

They're out of control. He's dripping snot. The dirty tissues are clutched in his hands. These wet balls of Kleenex. I saw one on the kitchen counter. I saw one on the kitchen floor, and someone had stepped on it, so it looked like a public restroom floor. Like what happens when there's urine-soaked paper inexplicably wadded up on the toilet floor. Tim's nose is dripping; his eyes are watering. He can't take allergy meds because they wipe him out, and he's a freakin' chemist, so he needs to be alert, and it's probably the dog who's causing everything. Tim's probably allergic to our new puppy, who we now have to keep—no matter what—but my husband is in tears over here.

And let me tell you this: I need him to keep his shit together, because someone has to attend to *my* shit, and if *his* shit is falling apart, I'm in trouble.

What do you think I'm going to do? Knock on my mother's door? *I think not.*

Plus, his tolerance for misery is so low. It's a goddamn runny nose. Try getting dosed with radiation. Try walking around with gray hair like an old man and asymmetrical implants (three separate friends sent me emails the other day on getting free tattooed areolas). At the end of the day, at the end of the tissue-expander-sleepless-night day, I am left with one breast clearly smaller than the other. Even my plans—my great plans—for body art are now skewed, rendered Picasso-esque.

Tim's allergies are freaking me out, and I'm still right there, behind him, tapping him on the shoulder, saying, *You're not attracted to me anymore. My pain will always, always be greater than yours. And what if your nose never stops running again? What will happen to the likes of us? To our dog, Snickers? To our status as Americans? Americans have dogs. This is something we talked about. But I sense it now, this turning away from me, this absence of you.*

Not even TV will save us.

I've been filled with anxiety.

* * *

Wendy.

I just registered Wendy for a two-night "camp" with a friend this spring. She leaves in a van; she has a sleeping bag; they have her insurance information, my phone number, Tim's phone number. It's a freakin' church group, it's only two nights, and I'm flipping out: *my baby, my baby.*

My firstborn possesses this thing that stresses me out, that I see and I respond to sharply, hoping to crush this part of her, this weakness I see in her. Wendy, thin-limbed, delicate, is a shadow-me, this other me, the Girl I No Longer Am. Wendy is easily hurt, eager to be liked, soft, so soft.

And it's almost like a joke, because who could ever imagine me like that, on the cusp of womanhood, breakable, teetering, such softness, such delicacy?

Tim can't.

When I tell him that I was like her, he doesn't see it: *You were never like that. Do you think she'd travel around Europe and Africa alone? Do you think she'd move to New York City alone?*

And I'm like, *She's me. She's me.*

That core of her, so easy to puncture, to injure.

What can we do to protect her heart? To make her stronger?

Tim once saw a strange child throw sand in Wendy's face: Wendy did not rise up. She did not rise up and fight. And how do I want my daughter to respond? Do I want her to turn the other cheek? Do I want her to kick some ass?

Yesterday, another child—*Dear Lord, these kids are bastards*—threw wood chips at Melody when she was going down the slide, and Wendy witnessed it. Wendy felt guilty for having seen it, for having allowed it to happen—and my anger soared. *Wendy,* I said, *you need to take care of this.*

I wanted to yell: *You need to step in. You need to tell that child that if she ever throws woodchips at my kid or any other kids, I will go batshit crazy and there will be teachers and parents and it will be ugly.*

Wendy, fragility aside, you tell this girl.

Wendy, gentle heart, you take care of this and you take care of it now.

And only then, after my anger had flared and she had wept, did I hold her.

I held her and I prayed aloud, because I knew—I knew—Wendy's guilt was bigger than any other injury done. My beautiful Wendy, with the trace of freckles on the bridge of her nose, sensitive to pain, sensitive to the complexity of emotions, instinctively sought forgiveness.

And, yes, of course, I want Tim to see, to see that our eldest daughter possesses this truly beautiful heart that if bruised too much, too often, will turn—not in the way he thinks. Wendy is shadow me, the Girl I No Longer Am.

The thought of Wendy crying unhinges me—makes me want to take my badass hair, my jean-clad-still-not-bad-butt to the front lines to protect her.

I am armed with a vicious tongue.

The grown-up woman is now a blazing rock-hard bitch. I will be a ballistic bitch. And am I protecting her from growing up? Am I protecting her from becoming me?

What can I do to preserve her loveliness?

* * *

Melody.

We have chosen sides, and it's not pretty.

Again, I'm like, *Tim, this isn't something you understand.*

Melody wants her Kidz Bop, her repetitive repertoire of artless pop songs. I remember my own repertoire, and the slow, mind-melding trick those promising love songs played on my Wendy-heart. By the time I hit adolescence, I was one of those hopeless romantics.

Ah, but Melody is different!

I just painted this picture of a vulnerable little girl, and Melody is something else, someone altogether *other*.

One crazy giveaway is her looks. Melody looks nothing like me. I wouldn't recognize her as my own daughter. There is no sign of me in her eyes, in her nose, in her mouth. She looks like baby Tim. I was left out of the blueprint. As far as I can tell, the only similarity we share is a disdain for instruction manuals, a low tolerance for riddles, and a prepubescent interest in popular music. And look where all that got me! I, so-called strong woman, shamelessly, perpetually, defer to Tim on all instruction manuals, all technical matters, any new home appliance.

(In truth, I'm playing dumb. I know I could look stuff up. But I don't want to. And Tim is a repository of useful information. Why must I know how to work the DVD player? And the riddles? Look, I've got better things to do with my time—as does Melody.)

But it's the pop music, the introduction of angst, the myth of romance, the bildungsroman narratives underlying the lyrics and feeding the ego, the id: Those are the shared interests that send me quaking, and what if Melody and I are ultimately linked in this: We find myths tantalizing?

What if we are co-heirs in the myth of romantic love?

What if we fall prey to the same stories, and Melody—possessing a beauty that was never mine—goes searching for the pretty boy, the bad boy?

How do I stop her, save her, spare her the pain of his charm?

And, please please *please* do not speak to me of smart phones in the hands of children, of iPods, iPads, tablets, and other bullshit which, supposedly, make them tech savvy. I see them as gateway drugs, as things pulling away my babies, revealing ugly secrets. I don't need my girls to type messages with their thumbs. Toss out the texting and throw them a book.

Oh, Melody is fortified with an ethereal beauty—a kind of beauty outside of my experience—but she seems to long for a connection to others that her poor mother longed for too.

What happens when such longing is found in a beautiful girl?

What disadvantage or advantage is beauty?

Melody is boisterous, lively, fiery, confident. She'll fight me. She'll throw a temper tantrum. But she'll stop; she'll listen; she'll absorb swan songs, Taylor Swift's rendition of the breakup, Adele's take on passion. She doesn't know what any of it means.

And I tell Tim, *Yet. She doesn't understand yet.*

What happens when my beautiful girl figures it out?

* * *

I've been filled with anxiety.

I blame our plunge into *Breaking Bad* for these exposed nerve endings, for my psychosis.

Ah, dear reader, you thought you were dealing with someone sane.

37

Remission (April 20, 2016)

One benefit of living next to your mother is that she can forewarn you about *every* outbreak of salmonella, *every* airbag defect, and *every* spreading disease. Really, I knew about the re-emergence of the whooping cough, the dangers of eating processed foods and drinking soda, and the hazards of not washing produce way before anyone else knew. As you might imagine, it was a *huge* surprise to discover that I had cancer.

It's technically under one year and I'm supposedly done with the disease, so do I change the title of the book?

(You know I still believe I'll die, right?)

Remission.

Both the medical oncologist and the radiation oncologist gave me speeches on remission.

"It's a state of mind."

"Some people get bored without the constant management and routine of treatment."

I thought, *They obviously don't have small children.*

"Now, you'll just need to get on with living."

I still see doctors, but not as frequently.

I have the option of going in for further reconstructive surgery to fix the small boob. Tim is for leaving it. And I don't know if this makes me happy or upset that he doesn't really care.

I'm on Tamoxifen for five years or more, which my medical oncologist seems to be a big fan of. "It's the best cancer drug out there." Even though it might cause uterine cancer and blood clots.

The hot flashes persist like nobody's business.

There you go. This is remission.

My guess is that I don't feel like you feel, however you might feel. I am not at peace; I wish I could say I were. I pretty much feel like a failure for acknowledging this. I have failed to have the positive attitude that will apparently infuse my being with healing; rather, I imagine that all of my skepticism, all of my years-in-the-making cynicism, will infuse my veins, course through my body, bring one of those remaining but quieted cancer cells on the fast-track to some other part of my body—which is ready and waiting, sown and plowed, like a garden with really good soil, ready for some serious metastasis. And when this happens, *it will all be my fault.*

Oh, ye of little faith!

Are you talking to me?

And then I think of my children. I think about seeing my time as finite, an allotment, and how I need to use it to savor moments with them, giving them a mother every second of their day. Being that mom, that mom they'll always carry with them, even if I die soon.

Again, I think: *I failed at this, too.*

I still get so mad at them. I still yell. The other day, I ruined their breakfast at Dunkin' Donuts because they didn't do something I said, and I got so mad that Melody had tears in her eyes. I apologized. I asked for their forgiveness. But still. I am their surviving mom.

This Bitch Lives!

If I die in a year or two or five, who will they remember?

Tim and I. *I don't know.* Maybe I'm too fragile to think too much about us.

Sometimes, I can think about our rampage of a history, and I can be really happy. We've landed here, and it's not a bad spot. Sometimes I think, *Wow! I have one of the best marriages I've ever seen! Crazy, but true, considering I'm hell and he's nuts!* How did it happen? How did we end up as such good friends, able to deal with each other's idiosyncrasies so expertly? How did we manage to give our kids this grace of a good time?

And, sometimes, I can think about us, about our tragic-comic path, and be very sad.

And then I have to stop writing.

I have been haunted by one of Tim's comments. I don't know how we got on the subject, but I know it wasn't during one of our purported "good times." He told me, "You don't live in the moment. You've never been more buried in your writing than you are now."

The truth of the matter is this: *He's right.*

My inclination, when cancer struck, was to write.

My inclination was not so much to survive as it was to write—but I want to be clear here: *I wanted to write for my children.*

That is what I would do for them. I'm not sure I can find the proper words to articulate this, but this is what I *can do* for my children.

While Tim may need my physicality, I wanted to be present, even more present than bodily present, by giving my children all that I have written.

This is me, girls.

This.

I love you.

Do not lose heart.

I write for you.

I'll see you in the next place.

But I'm in remission, which means, then, I need to be fully present in my life! I need to occupy my moments!

I need to occupy this body.

(I had this old "boyfriend"—I guess we can call him that—who said to me, accusatorily, "I'd rather live than write." He was a beach bum, into the ocean. I responded, "I write to live." Dramatic. Is this decades-old conversation somehow applicable?)

One of my creative writing students paraphrased Hemingway as saying that a writer is never present in any moment except when he or she is in war.

I can't find the quote anywhere, but it sounds right.

Writers—artists?—always exist outside of the moment. They are always removed from the present, hovering, tweaking reality to render it another way.

Is this true?

I think it is!

Remission, alas.

We're going to *Breaking Bad* the hell out of tonight.

38

Resting in Peace (May 5, 2016)

Now is not a good time to write. But, obviously, it's time to write.

I have tons of papers and student portfolios to grade (from that teaching career I feebly maintain).

But I've decided—despite anything I've previously said—that I'm going on antidepressants to try to stop the hot flashes in an effort, really, to sleep. Sleep and sleep and *sleep*. I think it's the hot flashes that are keeping me awake. Though it could also be the implants that prevent me from rolling onto my stomach. Or maybe I can't sleep because of the anxiety over my impending demise.

Rest in peace, Prince! I will miss you! Even though I didn't know you, owned only a smidgen of your music, and made fun of you a little bit when you renamed yourself "The Artist Formerly Known as Prince" (from 1993 to 2000—due to contractual reasons, it turns out). You were part of my life. What I mean is that I liked having you around. That whole "1999" thing: we were together back then, those early days. And your death felt like part of my generational structure being chipped away. Like I could look up at the top of Generation X Mountain, rocks falling on my head, and shout, "Landslide!"

How is this, in any way, related to my cancer memoir?

Well, it is, of course.

Drugs! Artistry!

So I'll try antidepressants.

I have been so adamant about not messing with what I have, that measure of artistic grace I have been given. So, yeah, I'm the one who is always clean and sober. I'm not messing with my chemistry.

I want my highs and lows, the volatility!

It fuels my writing!

But, yeah, I'm doing it.

I'll do it for the book! I think an antidepressant might "round out" my cancer experience. The next few months are pretty open for taking off the hard edges of my life.

And this whole thing makes me feel close to Prince!

May he rest in peace.

39

Experiment Over! (undated)

Y eah, it's over.

I thought I should tell you.

I took an Effexor last night at a low dosage, in order to combat hot flashes, in an effort to sleep. The antidepressants everyone can't wait to get me on.

Well, I had a super horrible reaction to the med. I took it at 8:40 p.m., right around the time Tim got home from a mountain-biking daytrip to Payson. I felt weird by the time I went to sleep. What followed was a sleepless night of dizziness, some nausea, and mega-anxiety.

I flipped out.

I started making plans for letting Tim sleep as long as possible so he could help me in the morning. He'd take care of the kids, he'd call my friends Raegan and Siobhan (both doctors). He'd get me to an ER to pump my stomach.

Damn: It's not gonna work.

I hope it works for you. I hate the loss of control, which might be wrongly connected to some skewed concept of personal autonomy.

I cling, desperately, pathetically, to self-sovereignty—and it'll be the death of me.

This is a prophecy.

When I thought about this at two, then three, and then four and five in the morning, I got insane. Paranoid. I couldn't get the drugs out of my system.

They're still there now!

All night long, I kept thinking about how my kids would be forever affected by the horror that is me because I'm unable to soften the blows of my vitriolic personality.

All of this on the heels of a very troubling conversation with Tim on Donald Trump, so he was in my head, too!

But I'm done. It's over.

40

Oh, No! The Political Post . . .
(May 9, 2016)

So, listen. I keep saying to people, "I don't talk politics. I'm apolitical." And then I keep talking politics.

As my husband aptly pointed out, "You have to choose your battles."

I need to shut up and remember my artistic agenda—whatever that is.

(But cancer eased up right when the political season heated up!)

Politics—at long last—is part of my writing landscape, my interior design. I can say this now. I've never fully reconciled my politics with my writing; I've only seen myself as abandoning one for the other.

Did cancer sharpen my perspective at all?

I've written very little about my former life in politics (ha!).

Now is the time!

The first thing you need to know is that I've met Hillary Clinton. And she likes Diet Cherry Coke. I've never met Donald Trump, though I've peed in the Trump Tower on Fifth Avenue dozens of times. When I was in grad school at NYU, his was the only bathroom open to the public that I could easily find in that part of Manhattan. Maybe that's a point for him.

This presidential campaign is freaking me out.

I need to go back in time . . . .

How I became a writer.

Why I cannot vote for Donald Trump.

There, I said it out loud. *I will not vote for Trump.*

For me to do so would be simply absurd, given my, um, political history.

It sounds nuts when I tell people I majored in political science in college because of U2, though I think it's true. Bono made me do it!

It was the aesthetic combo of art and politics, the white-flag raising, the solidarity they uniquely expressed between rock n' roll and Judeo-Christian principles. My own personal religious beliefs were rendered legitimate in rock n' roll terminology! This had never happened before, and it's never happened since—and this is why I will forever forgive U2 of any foibles, forever displaying my loyalty to them. We are brethren, so to speak. Sure, I'd sign that Amnesty International petition passed around at the concert. Sure, I'd participate in the human rights candlelight vigil. And you better believe I would not back down in my show of support for MLK.

So, yes, I got multiple degrees in political science, fully intent on a career in international relations—largely due to my love of U2.

(I still planned to write fiction on the side, I guess. Shark-story, still relevant.)

Life in New York: I think one could sum up my ideology by just looking at U2 and saying, "She's with them." I was, oddly, uncomfortably, a huge liberal with Christian beliefs. Liberalism combined with moral absolutes?

If Bono could do it, I could, too!

After college, I had three jobs in New York. First, I worked—of course—for Amnesty International, putting my U2-indoctrination to good use. Second, I worked at the United Nations Association-USA, a non-profit focused on U.S. involvement at the U.N. I remember encountering some scorn from churchy people who spoke of one-government conspiracies and the evils of internationalism. I offended people. Oh-the-fuck-well. Third, I landed at the Council on Foreign Relations. It was there that I met Hillary Clinton.

I need to be super honest here. These are sizzling hot credentials, but I sucked *completely*. I was a total failure. I lacked all ambition. I was never more than a glorified admin assistant.

I was twenty-five, living in Manhattan, and frankly, I didn't believe in it at all. It wasn't my Gen-X cynicism that separated me from the other political scientist peeps. We were *all* cynics. It was this: *I was uncomfortable with what seemed to me to be the quantification of topics that were predominantly matters of qualitative inquiry.* Game Theory—the main spiel in grad school—seemed dumb to me. We were talking world peace. We were talking saving the world. This was life-and-death stuff, the problem of evil. Philosophy! Religion!

I knew that I had to be a writer. I was a liberal arts girl.

I had to accept my student loan fate, abandon my career path, and embrace the absurdity of "being a writer."

I mean, if we were talking about saving the world, let's just admit this one small thing: Politics wasn't going to cut it.

What does a liberal do with her new decision to abandon a career in human rights to be a writer? She goes to South Africa with a backpack, ready to experience it all since Nelson Mandela was the leader, the first democratically elected president in post-Apartheid South Africa, of course! Nelson Mandela!

South Africa was formative, pivotal. There, my worlds meshed. The landscape, with its lush greens, rocky coasts, wild flora, unruly fauna, roll of clouds—all spoke to me, aesthetically. The clash of people, of black and white, First and Third World, old and new, rich and poor, stucco mansion and tin-can shanty town—all spoke to me, politically. It was the ultimate classroom for a political-science-nonprofessional-turned-struggling-writer. Such beauty amidst such suffering! I would write, focusing on this pinpoint, this meeting point or vortex at which good and evil met in a mess that is humanity.

So, yeah, I became a writer.

More school.

In an ugly irony, I found myself politically disaffected in my early marriage. Not only did I decide to forsake what I dismissed as mere political rhetoric, but I also dismissed all of politics.

For the first decade of my marriage, I stopped paying attention to the world.

I think, in retrospect, I might say I was preoccupied with my own unhappiness.

I reexamined conservatism, though. I embraced a new ideology: Individual hearts had to enact change; the government couldn't impose it.

This was a difficult time for me, so my lack of global concern is linked with an ugly myopia. I was a new mom, and I sucked at that, too. Tim and I fought all the time. (He once yelled at me, "If you love socialism so much, why don't you move to Canada?" I once called him a racist.) I listened to Dennis Prager a lot. I tried to enmesh myself in church. My old friends were—and continue to be—*baffled* by my newfound conservatism.

I felt disembodied, somehow.

The Dark Times dissipated, however.

This is a long, crazy story—family, marriage, personhood, church.

But, right about when U.S. politics were going batty, I woke up.

(Then I got cancer! Ha!)

I emerged in a rough spot but at peace, frankly. I was now established as a writer, albeit a not-very-successful one. People no longer even associated me with international relations. My marriage got good (we're still pretty different, though). I stopped listening to conservative radio and went back to NPR.

(Thank God!) We ended up switching to a new church that was markedly racially diverse. (This was not intentional on our part; however, it resulted in meeting a particular need for me: to have my Christianity mesh with my sense that all people are created equally. Hugely complicated, I would say that my liberalism and my conservatism finally made sense.)

But there has been displacement.

My seemingly inane conservatism put me at odds with the worlds in which I am most involved: the worlds of writers and artists and academics.

In short, I didn't fully fit in among the liberals and I didn't fully fit in among the conservatives. The crazy part is that both sides get a little mad at me. The liberals are angry at my betrayals; the conservatives—more cocky, by the way—consider me ignorant.

I've stayed right of center.

I embarrass my mom.

I hang out with both liberals and conservatives, more libs than conservatives.

I still can't understand why in the world anyone would think it's OK for us to have the right to carry guns into classrooms.

And I will not vote for Donald Trump.

It sounds a little to me like Pontius Pilate washing his hands when discussing the crucifixion of Christ, and saying, "My hands are clean."

It's a kind of cultural violence.

Can a memoir-in-real-time ignore the world at large? Should I blow off the world? Will my myopia be justifiable now?

I guess I see caring about politics as part of getting better; the world has become larger than my tumors. So I went nuts on Trump as I went into remission.

Good writing involves harnessing abstractions like Truth, Goodness, and Beauty, and rendering them concretely. Stories are concrete displays of abstractions. How can I, as a writer who once abandoned politics, say nothing?

All I can say is that this is a memoir in real time.

Life with cancer!

Isn't this what Tim wanted for me? To occupy the moment?

41

I Left the House (May 16, 2016)

I made it out of the house at night without Tim for the first time since the diagnosis in June 2015! A Prince Memorial at a club (the Crescent Ballroom) with friends! Yes, I left the club ridiculously early! No, I didn't get to see the actual musician I went to see (the rumor flying around was that she'd hit the stage at 11 p.m.)! Yes, I slept very poorly that night! Yes, the kids were up and flying from the rafters when I got home!

But it was fun.

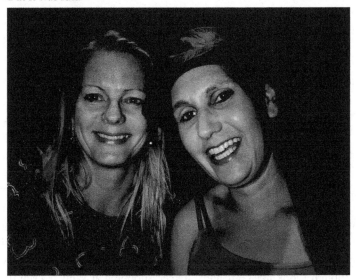

This is my great friend, Odette. She's Dutch. We don't deserve her.

42

Moving On (May 22, 2016)

Things have been rough. I guess I keep complaining.

What do people expect? Chemo ends, radiation ends, the hair starts coming in . . . . Should I be doing some kind of happy dance?

First, there's this: I'm not over it. And it feels, like it *really* feels, as if everyone else is ready to move on.

Second, now I'm dealing with my inner bitch. Interestingly enough, while I think my husband really wanted me to come to terms with her in our early marriage and I felt mostly vindicated for my behavior then, THIS is the time that I feel like it's me—my problem, my shit, my horribleness.

I'm the bitch, and I'm doing the damage.

Third, people keep wanting me to take drugs, except my mom, who needs them herself.

Fourth, my haircut! How dumb is that?

So, yeah, I'm just not ready to move on—and it's been causing some tension in the house. In my marriage. Like I'm just not so sure that I'm going to live, so I'm not really wanting to plan for a future with me in it.

When we look at our finances, this is what I see: I need to make sure that my girls are OK, and I'd like to keep them in a private school, so let's direct our money towards their tuition. My girls have sweet friends who don't do meth or talk about blow jobs, and my daughter's fourth-grade teacher is awesome, even though I know she'd hate me if she read my books, so, if I die, I'd l like them at their school. In the meantime, I'll keep buying my clothes at Kohl's even though I look like crap, and I'll keep shopping at WinCo, even though

Tim makes fun of my upper-middle class childhood which didn't really involve places like WinCo, and it's true that WinCo's produce is a little gross.

But a deal's a deal.

When we look at our finances, this is what Tim sees: Maybe we should think about remodeling the house or trading in his Nissan, which we don't even like. The girls are getting to be that age—you know, *that age*—at which they'll remember our life. Plus, he hates that master bedroom. So, let's knock some walls down, maybe. Build an addition. The girls can each have their own room? Why aren't I watching that remodeling show with them? Even my plastic surgeon keeps it playing on repeat all day long in his waiting room (as if it's a metaphor for possessing a beautiful future). It's a good show! Those people have a knack; they have vision! We could open this place up, and still keep grandma happy behind the bookshelf! I'll get a job now, too. Right? We're not talking about pulling them out of their school. I'm going to work more, yes? Back to full-time, yeah?

And I'm like, *Yeah, if I'm not dead.*

Yeah, so, my cancer card has been officially revoked, and I'm no longer supposed to be keeping this cushy schedule in which I teach my two community college classes—and then read or write until the girls come home and I become a full-time crappy mom. Look, I'm fine with working. I really am. I understand that we need it, that we've made costly education decisions, that my writing brings in *nothing*.

Part of me is grateful that Tim is thinking about a future with me.

Another part of me is thinking, *Not so fast! I'm gonna die!*

And there are marital woes, frankly. Now that the urgency has subsided, we've maybe relaxed a little. It's been tough on me to see his urgency give way.

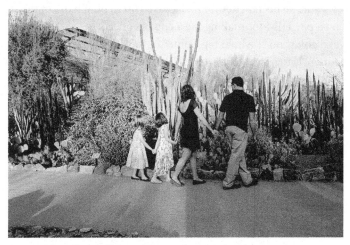

Photo by Lex Treat, photographer. Used with permission.

Tim said of that picture, not meanly, "I lost her."

And it's true. What an irony of life, too: You only know you had it when it's gone!

"Well, she's not coming back," I responded.

Yes, my inner bitch is thriving. Chemo killed a lot, but it didn't kill her.

And what of my toxicity? What effect will it have on my children? Tim and I, for better or worse, have learned to navigate each other's minefields. We do so in highly imperfect ways. I think our children have witnessed a lot of bad things, but they've seen a lot of good things, too: they've seen us stay together when no one thought we would, they've seen us laugh together a lot, they've seen us cuddling on the couch, they just learned that we've had sex more than two times (once for each of them). But I worry about the other things we've taught them, the things I've taught them. With my irritation, my own persistent urgency. I worry incessantly about ruining their sweetness.

Get thee on drugs!

I look very much like a boy, too. And I hate that. I'm not dealing well with it. Tim said, "I thought you handled baldness better than this."

My looks are hitting me hard. I bought some cute little lingerie thingy, but you know what I think when I see it with the tags still on? I think, *What's the point?*

Briefly, in cancer news:

I went to ONE physical therapy appointment and cancelled the next one. All of the therapists looked so damn sporty and like personal trainers, and the place looked like a gym, so I thought I'd rather stay home and read my book.

I had a Groupon for a massage, and I went—picking the worst one EVER. It would've been better if I had asked Tim to punch me in the stomach and then I'd pay HIM for making me a cup of coffee.

We're going on a whole big family outing to my next oncologist's appointment on Thursday to determine if I'll start getting monthly Lupron shots to inhibit estrogen production. I'm leaning towards them.

43

Zootopia (June 23, 2016)

I write from Flagstaff, Arizona, where we are vacationing (no Disney this year!), having met our beloved friends, Penny and Brian, who came down from Seattle. Tim bikes. I drink coffee and write. My girls play with Penny and Brian's kids. We meet up later and say deep things based on years of crazy friendship. We've already discussed *Zootopia*, which they see as a parable of sorts on transgendered stuff/biology-is-not-destiny and we see as a tale on how the lion and the lamb will dwell together.

We've already argued over politics. At Chick-fil-A. Dear Lord, I said it aloud. (Where's the Hobby Lobby in Flagstaff?)

But back to *Zootopia*. I loved it!

Freakin' Democrat!

But, cancer. Back to the cancer. This is about me dying of cancer.

I used henna on my hair. Forget everything I said about sticking with the gray. I'm sticking with the red.

I'm doing a little organic/paraben-free frenzifying around here, too. Forget everything I said about kale and not buying into this naturopathic mumbo-jumbo, too. I'm detoxifying our lives. A little. I bought the girls organic deodorant, even though they don't stink yet. Sunscreen, henna, lotion. That sort of thing.

YOU'RE NOT GOING TO BELIEVE THIS PART. I read some random article on how tart cherry juice helps insomniacs sleep. I bought some. Organic, of course. *And it works!* I can't believe it myself. A doctor-friend said it apparently boosts the body's own natural production of melatonin. I just switched to capsules, rather than the juice (because, well, *sugar feeds cancer*). Guess what. *It still works.* Surely, this won't last.

(Note from the future: It didn't last.)

I had my first OB/GYN appointment since the cancer diagnosis. I hadn't been there since that day that Tim and I showed up, mere wreckage, unannounced, asking to see my gynecologist so that he could explain this cancer to us. This latest appointment was uneventful, but still I felt that wreckage right there with me.

I found out that I have a UTI infection, which pretty much surprised me because I didn't feel like I had one—and I usually know it. Why didn't I know? Cherry juice?

I'm going to begin getting Lupron shots in July. These shots inhibit estrogen production, and they're only newly being used to treat breast cancer—so it's a bit of an unknown. Not everyone is opting for this. I am.

And I met one of my former chemo nurses, Karen P., for coffee. I told her it was for my book.

I'm always wiped out—like stumbling-fool exhausted—by around 10 p.m.

I think I'm an introvert now, and I always billed myself as an extrovert. I personally think my introversion began a while ago, pre-cancer. I withdrew earlier. First, when my marriage was falling apart and no one seemed to get it. Then, when my marriage wasn't falling apart and I felt older, more like being a writer, inclined to fully submerge myself in my eccentricities, and only interested in talking to Tim.

I'm really so irritable post-cancer.

When wasn't I edgy? *I have always been irritable.*

I do feel, however, a little more responsible for my irritability now.

I grew up in an irritable milieu; *the women were good, but irritable.*

Now, I wonder at that, more than I previously did. Perhaps I should stop the cycle. Lest my girls become irritable women as well. Right now, I'm one of those moms whose kids know she loves them, though she yells at them a lot. This is the way it goes in our clan. I was raised the same way. I don't want to do that anymore. I'd like to stop. The state of irritability was there long before the malignant cells multiplied; the brush with death made me more responsible.

I'm trying Prozac soon. Even though I said no more antidepressants ever. I got a prescription, under the pretense of wanting to address the hot flashes—which I do want to address, though I have ulterior motives. Maybe I'll be a better mom. I have the Prozac at home, waiting. I'll try it around the Fourth of July. I'm waiting till I don't have a lot of obligations, lest I flip out like I did with my last antidepressant attempt.

154

Actually, I feel as if I'm in some kind of holding tank, waiting for the clichés to take hold: the bomb to drop, the shoe to fall. That cancer in my one lymph node? You know it escaped. That nodule on my lung? I never had Valley Fever. (I have another scan on July 1.) All this radiation I've had? That can't be right. *The. Shoe. Will. Drop.*

But remission, I suppose, is a good time to get in touch with my emotions (go on Prozac), take charge of my body (henna), reconnect with my husband (*Sons of Anarchy* sucks so badly), get involved in the community (fight with friends over politics), read more Elena Ferrante (yay!), get a job (Tim told me that as long as no one's paying me for my writing, it's a hobby—so I better find a way to bring in some income), detoxify our lives (switch to pine-pellet cat litter), figure out our sex life (I still haven't written about this, have I?), work on selling my unpublished novel (it's complicated and I'm sad, but really, what else will I do if not author books no one reads?), be grateful (my girls are great kids, and I think my marriage is better than yours—though I keep having to tell this to Tim, who doesn't believe it), try to be nicer to my mom (who was going to be the subject of my next book and who, undeservedly, bears much of my heartache), and meet up with my old chemo nurse, Karen (she'll later defriend me on Facebook over Trump).

So, we're technically at about the one-year cancer mark, which renders my title obsolete. The tattoos, still happening, will be in January 2017—though nothing is scheduled. Right now, remission.

Doesn't *remission* sound to you like *not now, but later*? I like *cancer-free* quite a bit, though it sounds like a lie.

44

Back to the Writing Life
Final Notes (July 2016)

I told Tim, "I hate my hair so much."
He said, "Put a bird on it."

* * *

Organic deodorant seems to mean B.O.

* * *

I took ten milligrams of Prozac a day for three days. I doubled it to twenty. I was supposed to ease into my twenty, just in case I flipped out. I upped it again. Thirty.

Tim anxiously awaits my kindness. *Bitch Be Gone.*

I eagerly anticipate not being able to fry an egg on my forehead.

I really need for you to understand one thing clearly and explicitly: *When a woman says she's hot-flashing, it's no joke.*

I texted Tim at work yesterday: *I def feel something with more Prozac. Not sure what.*

Tim responded: *Happiness?*

I texted back: *You wish.*

Apparently, my Diva-Bitch Personality is *stronger* than one of the most common psychiatric drugs in modern medical history.

Two months and then I'm done. (Writing from the future: It didn't work. I'm off all antidepressants.)

* * *

I had a PET Scan to look at the nodule on my lung. It's not cancer!

* * *

Things I've Learned from Facebook About Being a Writer:

1. Dr. Seuss's first book was rejected twenty-seven times.

2. Stephen King's *Carrie* was rejected thirty times.

3. Margaret Mitchell's *Gone with the Wind* was rejected thirty-eight times.

4. Arrogance looks a lot like confidence, and you can't be arrogant, but you must be confident.

5. That said, you gotta be humble, but all the while you must self-promote because no one else will promote you, except your mom. *No one else.*

6. Everyone wants to write a book.

7. Everyone is writing a book.

8. Everyone thinks he or she can write a book.

9. Everyone has this fabulous story that you should write because it's a guaranteed bestseller.

10. No money coming in? *That's Because You Don't Work.*

11. There are a lot of crappy books out there.

12. There are a lot of great books out there.

13. Most people are not readers of literature, and I'm so sad.

14. I'm not Dr. Seuss.

15. I'm not Stephen King.

16. I'm not Margaret Mitchell.

17. I overdramatize my life.

18. I don't care that I overdramatize my life.

19. Writers love being writers, no matter what they say.

20. The trick is to find some kind of Zen-like balance between self-publicity and displays of humility. I have no clue how to do this.

21. Facebook really is perfect for failing writers, though one tends to annoy many, many people.

22. I'm supposed to hate Amazon, but I don't.

23. EBooks and audiobooks are OK.

24. Do not ask your friends if they've read your books, if they own your books, or what they think of your books.

25. You're only as good as your last book.

* * *

Phoenix + Tamoxifen = Raging hot flashes.

Guys, they're *debilitating.*

Spontaneous public humiliation, anywhere, anytime. With friends. With acquaintances.

Phoenix is unbearable, like hell, like a lava pit, like a scene in *Lord of the Rings*—the Gollum parts.

A sex life is, um, problematic. Sweaty bodies colliding? Are you kidding me?

Tim has said, "I feel a little bad about asking you to get a job." Picture me in front of a class, drenched, going over the syllabus, the freshmen all nervous.

I look like I just ran a marathon.

I've hot-flashed mid-workout, on a treadmill. I've just plodded through, wondering if I might faint.

Hugging my kids? A problem.

Cat on the lap? A problem.

Yes, I'm drinking a lot of water.

* * *

At what point would you stop the life-saving drugs for quality-of-life issues? I try to preserve my life mostly for my children and my husband. What if I can never touch them again? What if my life post-cancer is about sitting still under a fan?

In all honesty, I'm overwhelmed. And desperate. I'd have a surgical procedure to end the hot flashes. I'll relent on my drug-abstention and try anything.

I could stop the Tamoxifen and Lupron altogether.

* * *

Should I die, these are my last wishes:

1. Tim should re-marry. I've told him my personal choice for a new wife, which did make for an awkward conversation. I need a good woman who will love my kids and take care of him. But, second wife, I will tell you this: *He's not what you think he is, but he's a good guy.*

2. I'm going to call on Penny to explain my death to my kids. Not over and above Tim, but beside him. Sadly, I don't think I'm the first woman to ask this of her, which must say something pretty amazing about her.

3. Cremate me.

4. Take care of my mom.

5. Tim doesn't like my cats, but he should keep them *indoors*.

6. If my third novel isn't published, get it published.

7. If people would like to send donations somewhere, I choose Food for the Hungry.

* * *

I leave you with a cliff hanger. *Will I live, or will I die?*

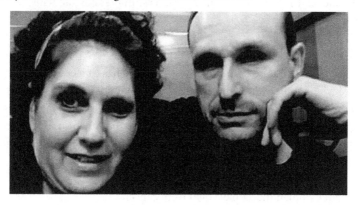

An Epilogue (May 31, 2019)

I write now, nearly three years later.

There is a surprise ending.

I shared a draft of this epilogue (now kaput) with Penelope Krouse, my friend and first reader. She said, "My general impression, actually, is one of anxiety."

I'm, like, *Uh-oh.*

I'm also, like, *Um, yeah???*

How else does one end a book in which one has cancer?

Maybe another kind of woman, another kind of writer, will leave her readers with a sense of peace. Where, after all, is this Christianity business that pops up periodically throughout my tome—too much so for the secular, too little for the saints? Haven't I found peace? Haven't I come to some understanding of the sovereignty of God and the nature of predestination?

Better women than I exist out there.

Better women than I have died from cancer.

I can only offer you a wicked brew of peace and anxiety. *Penny, I've always been less faithful than you.*

* * *

In the foreword, I mentioned that this was originally a private blog that unfolded in real-time. I do want to say a little something about that. My revisions had very little to do with content. Perhaps the biggest revision was that I had to dump vast amounts of political ranting. I really went ballistic over the election season, losing, incidentally, friends—many of whom were among those in the supportive cancer crowd.

This was emotionally difficult for me—to be so embraced while ill, to feel so fiercely about an issue apart from my health, and to experience disdain over my views (I admit that the disdain was mutual). I might offer a gross comparison. After a person is wounded, there is a crumbly scab. Dried blood shielding the one-time open sore. Even though scabs can be revolting, they are marks of healing. Maybe, just maybe, my political rampage implies the healing of a wound.

Politics, my scab.

Finally, I was able to look outward rather than inward.

Might I suggest that this is the first of my peace offerings? If only for a flickering second, I was able to transcend myopia, my preoccupation with self, my blatant self-absorption—to, still true to character, immerse myself OBSES-SIVELY in a world beyond my breasts? I was, finally, able to think of the world my children may inherit without me.

So I went crazy on politics.

However, I want to begin my epilogue by thanking the cancer crowd. Even those who were later turned off by my liberal politics. Thank you for reading my unedited cancerous prose. How does one support a writer? One reads the writer's stuff! I thank you people first.

And now I'll get to the good stuff, the surprise ending. Maybe.

* * *

I'm now considered cancer-free. I see anywhere from one to four doctors a "season." (Maybe zero appointments in February and three in May, or two in December and six in July—I've been on a school schedule for my whole life.) I'm always seeing an oncologist or a general practitioner or getting a scan. I worry a lot about the radiation. I'm perpetually high strung. I'm really not bitter. I don't think I'm depressed. I'm not on antidepressants. I am an insomniac on sleep meds, which means I get tired easily and early. I think I'd be considered rather active and energetic—but it all falls apart by 6 p.m. I have borderline high blood pressure and borderline high cholesterol now, which I never had before. I never stayed on the Lupron, though I may try it again; I gained weight on it. I've been on Tamoxifen for years now, and the hot flashes persist. They are—quite simply—the WORST part of this whole thing.

Hot flashes warrant separate chapters and chapters and chapters. All I can say is that they are constant, uncomfortable, embarrassing, and alienating, and they effectively make human contact miserable.

I have tried many, many things to combat them. I went nuts on Effexor. Prozac didn't do shit. Vitamin E did nothing. Amberen, nada. Peridin-C, nope. Black Cohosh isn't good for me because it may promote estrogen-production. Queen Bee Pollen was a no-go.

I never tried acupuncture. I should.

If there is anything ruining my life, it is this.

I pretty much work full-time again, irregularly, as an adjunct prof on multiple campuses. That unpublished book came out, and I think it is *The Big Deal That Wasn't*. I manage to be a writer too—and I owe a lot to Tim, who has made my writing life possible.

Doctors may not tell you this part. Urinary urgency. Someone told me that cancer people, post-chemo, often have an urgency to pee. I was surprised—but not *that* surprised. I just thought it was me! It's controllable, though I once wet myself at a Mary Poppins play and it was utterly humiliating (I'm surprising myself by including this detail)—and I started wearing sanitary napkins in public for a few months. I no longer do; I just pee every five seconds. I've heard it's debilitating for some women. No doctor ever mentioned this to me. Everyone in my family thinks I'm crazy for going to the bathroom so much. Really, I'm just afraid of the Mary Poppins fiasco.

I insist (probably delusionally) that I never had "chemo-brain." This is a chemo-induced foggy, not-super-sharp state of mind. *Listen, motherfuckers, I wrote two books during cancer.*

Even though I just called you all motherfuckers, I'd say that I'm considerably less irritable now—like it dissipated (in part). My daughters are eleven and thirteen. There's a lot of drama in the house. I'm on them often. They talk back; they always want to be on tablets or laptops; they don't do chores. That said, we're all really close.

I guess that it would actually be fair to say that—BY FAR—the second biggest lifestyle change (besides hot-flashing) has been my transformation from extrovert to introvert. And my introversion has meant that those three people—Tim, Wendy, and Melody—are my *world*. I very rarely step out without them, and this is atypical of my life before cancer. I *like* being home with them. I'm super dependent on Tim, and I don't give a crap what this says about me as a woman. I gather my kids in like a mother hen. I'm perfectly content staying home with them. There are unpleasantries associated with this new-found introversion: Tim and I are considered antisocial and I guess we are; my daughters aren't really exposed to all the benefits of a social life or church potlucks or big picnic get-togethers (and my kids *do* feel the lack), I feel that my own idiosyncrasies have been sharpened rather than tempered, and—maybe most significantly—I know that my "truest self" is only expressed in the company of three, and maybe that's bad. Or good.

Our family now takes epic road trips. I'm serious. Epic.

* * *

Look, here it is: My sex life is a mess.
Tim and I are beyond the body.

162

We are beyond little things, like sex.

We're on an astral plane (whatever that is) and our souls are cosmically aligned in this blissful union made up of a complicated past, multiple dependents, obligatory words, fart jokes, loyalty to *The Office*, more or less shared convictions, and oddly compatible senses of humor. I need him. He needs me. Our love is deep and it's complex.

I wouldn't even want to start over. *No interest whatsoever.*

Tim's too vested, too.

(Tim read an early draft of this epilogue and said I have it wrong. *Whatever.*)

Sex is affected by cancer. I do not think I'm alone in thinking this. In truth, no doctor has ever really addressed it with me. None. Close friends kinda lump post-cancer sex problems with middle-age/married sex problems. Medicine warnings and cancer websites talk about plummeting libido and menopause shit. A couple books I read made everything seem A-OK!

I'm finding, as I write, a hesitancy to share details. I apologize. I am unable to tell you that my body is anything but a betrayal.

* * *

I have learned this too: Autonomy is a myth we live by.

* * *

I had a second reconstructive surgery in November 2016. The small boob was opened along the scar and a new implant was put in there. The operation was a success. Radiation had hardened the previous implant, and it had shrunk into a weird, tiny boob.

I think there are disturbing jokes about weird, tiny appendages.

The talking mole in *Austin Powers*.

* * *

In January 2017, I went to the ER.

My breast scar became inflamed and itchy. I was admitted to the hospital for two nights with a staph infection. There was fear that I might lose the entire implant!

Are you fucking kidding me?

(But, if I lost it, would I be able to sleep again?)

The boob was saved by intravenous antibiotics. Or, as I like to put it, *I had a three-day vacation.* I had nonstop CNN to feed my political obsession. Van Jones, Anderson Cooper, Christiane Amanpour. Back to Van.

I speed-walked around the hospital floor listening to Trevor Noah's *Born a Crime*—I associate this hospital stay pleasantly with cutie pie Trevor Noah.

I had food on demand. Mediocre coffee. New socks. A big-ass water cup, dishwasher safe. Omelets and fresh fruit.

Plus, the nurses loved me—*loved* me—because I was no hassle whatsoever: just a mom taking a breather in a room with Trevor Noah and a filet of salmon. I was their favorite patient!

Tim and the kids visited for one hour in the evenings, the implant was fine, and I got all caught up on the news.

The only craziness? Tim pretty much fed the kids on taquitos from the gas station.

There was one sad, sad consequence from this staph infection business: *Tattoos were declared out!*

All of my plans for transforming my body into art: out.

I could risk it, but the puncturing of the skin is just that: a risk. And so, along with my other bodily failures, there is this one. I would have Barbie Doll Breasts Forever. No tribal tattoos, no vines snaking down my stomach, no blossoms disguising rips in the flesh.

No body art.

In other words, that aesthetic claim I was so eager to make? I couldn't make it.

* * *

Tim and I are together still, almost fifteen years.

Did I mention that we had a mix tape playing during our wedding reception that included the Eagles singing, "I've got a peaceful, easy feeling"?

That seemed, for so long, like a sick joke we were playing on ourselves.

But, now, I really do have a peaceful, easy feeling about my lover and my friend.

I'm not sure that Tim would put it this way, but I think our marriage has been marked by times in which I've held him up without wavering, and times in which he has held me up without wavering. Intense times. Now, partners in crime, keepers of the same secrets, intimates and best friends, we find ourselves ironically doing what we naively set out to do: Our happy marriage attests to the surety of our faith.

* * *

But we end in butchery.

The onslaught of the perfect body.

This plague of physicality.

I had believed I was beyond this onslaught and its sorrows.

I had believed I was immune to this kind of shame.

I believe that what happens next was tainted by my status of mom to girls. Thoughts about my body, the fate of my body . . . these things are influenced by my daughters.

I think back on my own girlhood—the U2 strung-out teenager, the lovelorn college girl, the faux New Yorker. The times when physical beauty was the ultimate. When boys' eyes might breeze over my body, its curves and slopes, and move along or not. When I acquired the habit of following eyes, the eyes of others, and it would make me both a careful observer (good for writing) and one who is damned to solemnity (bad for the soul: judgmental? hyper-perceptive?).

The onslaught of the perfect body is about the sadness of rock n' roll songs, the solace of pets, the temptation of gluttony, the reign of melancholy.

Now, in my own negotiations, I watch my girls—bombarded by idols—and I am reminded of the tyranny of image.

I remember the internal sighs, the spiritual cringing, the perpetual comparison of self to others.

* * *

Big family vacation in the middle of July 2017.

Always with the vacations.

My husband's family *really* loves New England.

Boston first. How could you not adore Boston? MFA, the Freedom Trail, the Commons.

The White Mountains in New Hampshire seemed terribly *Dirty Dancing* to me, complete with a resort that held ice-cream socials, a lake with paddle boats, and a questionable name. Indian Head. (Tim privately said to me, "Would 'Jew's Head' ever be OK?")

Here's a weird piece of trivia: Apparently, right on the highway at Indian Head, in 1961, an interracial couple, civil rights activists(!), were abducted by aliens. Barney and Betty Hill. Alien abductees.

I love this!

Flintstone-related?

Hampton Beach was where it finally happened.

There are two kinds of people in the world: *those who love the beach and those who do not.* Alex Gregory has a cartoon of a guy trying to talk on his cellphone on the beach. The caption is: "I'm sorry. I can barely hear you with this goddamn ocean behind me."

I resolved to quietly endure a full day in the sand. They did Boston for me. Indian Head offered up its funky charms. I'd do the beach. I would just put on my bathing suit, which looked okay with my fake-modest C boobs, slather on the SPF 5,000,000 sunscreen, grab my Barbara Kingsolver book (oh, Siobhan, an exquisite slog of a book!), sit next to a sister-in-law (two were there), wear an unattractive floppy hat, spy on my kids as they played with cousins, and let it happen. This was their day, not mine. *Really, Tim.* I was thinking, *I hate this. I love you guys. You better have fun.*

I lamented my decidedly unsexy look to Tim, "Oh *no*! Look at me."

"What?" he said. "You look like a nice, middle-aged woman."

Score?

Thank you?

I made it five hours on the beach. *Five. Hours.*

* * *

We were still at Hampton Beach, July 2017.

That afternoon, back in the room, after I ate leftover fried cod—kids still frolicking—my cancered breast scar was, well, a tad red. Reddening in an increasingly alarming way. Feeling a little enflamed. Maybe itchy?

Should I tell Tim or not?

I told him.

I had to.

So we went to the Urgent Care after I showered in what would be my last shower for two weeks.

I was still in blasé mode. "I just need an antibiotic and I'll go see my doc when I get home," I told the Urgent Care staff. "It's no big deal."

Interestingly, the Urgent Care went with this. They gave me Bactrim.

That night, hard-core, bone-chilling fever.

Combined with pain.

I mean, I was in *pain*.

I pulled the covers up to my chin in the Hampton Beach hotel room and shivered violently.

"Maybe it's septic," Tim said. "Let's just get in the car and drive to the hospital near my parents' house. *Right now*." It was nine o'clock at night. We were about an hour and a half away from Townsend, their adorable hometown in Massachusetts.

"No, I'm fine," I said, trembling from underneath the quilt. "I just need to sleep. The meds have to kick in." I was suddenly exhausted. "Go take the kids to see the fireworks."

I'll admit it now: This was my mistake.

We should've gone to the hospital immediately.

In the morning, I was immediately admitted to UMass Memorial in Leominster in time to watch O.J. Simpson's parole hearing. He was let out. They let him go. My scar unexpectedly ruptured in the table after an ultrasound. A hole opened up like all of those stories about the earth breaking and swallowing people. Brown liquid oozed from an open wound, and parts of it seemed globular. One could look into the chasm of my boob and see the implant—which was still intact

I was hospitalized in Massachusetts for two nights. Infectious disease doctors, doctors from nearby hospitals, a beautiful nurse from Zimbabwe who was only twenty-six. *Wooster* this, *Lemonster* that. An IV in my arm. No Trevor Noah. The food was not as good as it was in Scottsdale, but I sorta got a good vibe from the care. Tim was on the phone with my Arizona doctor, who did not want for me to get on a plane with an open wound.

It just happened.

They took it out.

At 10 p.m. on a Friday night. The doctor was from Worchester (*Wooster*) and he was the only one in the area.

It was gone.

No mourning period. I only had time to be upset about robbing my kids of the rest of the trip.

That's it.

No Ba-Da-Bing.

There is no Ba-Da-Bing.

Surprise ending: There are no Ba-Da-Bing Boobies.

* * *

I flew home with a very messed up body.

My plastic surgeon in Phoenix—top-notch, remember—was not pleased with the stitchery. Frankly, I think it was fine: a philosophical difference, a tension between Small Town and Big City medicine. I went in for a second surgery upon our return to clean it up and re-stitch it in time to start teaching in the fall semester.

Only one fake boob left.

Once you see it, you cannot un-see it.

Trust me on this.

* * *

We will build again.

That's what my Top-Notch Plastic Surgeon said.

This time, they would build a boob (like Build-A-Bear!) from my stomach or my butt or my thigh or my back. No foreign bodies. My own meat only.

* * *

Reader, I did not do it.

I've thought about going ballistic here, railing against the plastic surgery industry. Letting you know about the high incidence of failure in reconstructed breasts. Advising my girls to never fall for its trickery. Why had I bought into this body mythology? *What does any of this have to do with living?*

Rather, I'll just quietly tell you: *I do have regrets.*

But it's too late now.

* * *

I saw U2 with the girls in September 2017. Tim refused to go. "I'm done." My childhood best friend, Laura Cerny-Ciaccio, joined us. And this was fitting in every single way. I made a massive production out of the event, announcing my retirement from rock n' roll, and Tim fretted about me staggering through a stadium of stoned kids.

Everyone there was my age.

U2 was amazing.

I drove.

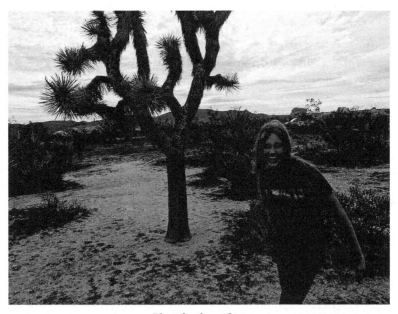

Photo by the author.

* * *

And then there were none.

I removed the left, remaining implant on December 2017. I timed it very carefully. I stopped teaching about a week earlier. Tim dropped me off at the surgeon's, and picked me up with a blueberry scone and a cup of coffee afterwards—like an old pro.

Neither of us even addressed the look of my flesh. I will tell you that it is not pretty. It is fleshy on one side, and tight as a drum on the other. Deformed. It looks like a botched job, for sure.

This time, we didn't sit around and mourn, or heave and ho. Rather, we persisted in our nightly binge of "Justified." We even went out for breakfast at IHOP the next day while the kids were at school.

I turned forty-eight.

I had prosthetics on within two hours of removing the drains.

* * *

I went alone to the specialty store for mastectomy bras. It's just you and this Jewish grandma in a fitting room in a tasteful boutique. You're in the room with Barbara. Barbara is her name, her *real* name. (*Why not name her?*) She fits you, stuffing your bra cups with prosthetics, tightening your straps. You pick the size. I stuck with my usual, *modest C, please.* Barbara pulled silk and satin from cubbies and compartments. Barbara brought out nighties and gowns.

And I was thinking, *Who could ever do a better job at this than a Jewish grandma? Is Barbara, like, the perfect person for this miserable job?* She brings out a bra for your deformities, adjusts it carefully, and declares, "Oh! You're so beautiful! Such a beautiful girl!"

She says it over and over—and it might be the last time you ever hear it.

You're such a beautiful girl.

You're such a beautiful girl.

* * *

May I confess that one of the hardest things I've ever done is something that I only did in January 2018? I didn't even tell Tim because I knew he wouldn't get it.

It took me till January 2018 to clean out my bra drawer. I opened it up and pulled out lace bras, underwire bras, black and magenta bras, a freakin' leopard-striped number, a veritable peep show of dainties. Who was this woman with these crazy props? Who did she think she was?

169

And why had I saved them? Why had I never tossed them out? Did I believe in some other kind of resurrection of the dead?

I put them all in a plastic trash bag and took them to Goodwill.

* * *

I love that damn dog.

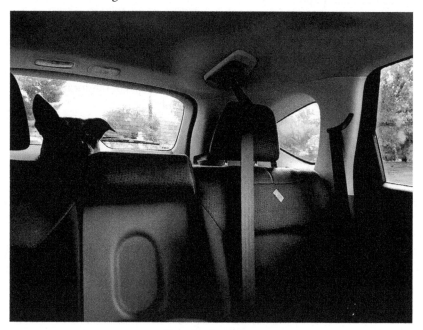

Photo by the author.

* * *

Philosophically, my body and my soul are in a kind of gnostic war. I struggle, in my disrepair, with hatred of the body, hatred of the physical world. The stuff of the soul must surely be the only good thing, yes? My soul, my soul: It is intact. I insist, *It is intact.*

And what is a woman but a soul in a physical casing? Is my womanhood any less than it once was? Is my womanhood under siege? Is this why they use that absurd rhetoric and call it "battling" cancer and "surviving"?

But listen: *I am not a gnostic.* I reject it. I believe in bodies, in reaching out, in touching earth, in running fingers through the fine and tangled hair of little girls, even in stepping in the grainy sand at the beach. The physical world matters.

But what place has my soul?
My battle, then, is unresolved.

* * *

Is there no redemptive end, then? Isn't it enough for it to be redemptive for you? Must it be so for me? I am content in writing like this, in giving myself away, exposing my body and its crimes—for you.

I offer that gift, a last peace offering.

That is my redemptive end: I affirm, completely, my willingness to use my own life as a palette, pens instead of paint, the canvas of my body, to tell you this story about what it's like.

And now, with the remains of my stitched flesh, all tattered in red and pinched with extra folds—Frankensteinian again, alas, forever—I ask how might my monstrosities fit in?

Written on the body, indeed.

Body betrayer, of course.

My true self. My truest self. Emerging. Refusing the façade, the pretty.

I see a narrative. I see a story. Did I just shred my flesh for the drama of it, my life a canvas, my breasts real pockets full of metaphoric posies?

I wrote another love story, yes?

If I stop at this moment, have I written the redemptive end?

Appendix

The cute kid quotes I couldn't use but promised to put in the book . . .

Wendy

1. Both girls were petting Jules, the cat. Wendy told Melody, "One of us has to go away, and it's you."

2. When Wendy saw Bosco, our cat, she'd call, "Bosis! Bosis!" She'd toddle after him and say, "I wanna love him." She'd touch his back. "I wanna be gentle." She'd ring her fingers around his tail. "I wanna be quiet. I wanna be nice."

3. Wendy heard me say to Bosco, "He's a good boy." Tim came into the room, and Wendy announced, "It's Daddy. He's a good boy."

4. I asked Wendy, "What's your stuffed ostrich's name?"
She answered, "Duck."

5. One day, something was floating in her lemonade. I asked, "What is it?"
She said, "Maybe a booger."
I said, "I doubt it."
Wendy responded, "It must be a cucumber."

6. She asked, "Where does the poop go when you flush the toilet?"
I told her about waste management facilities.
Wendy responded, "That's a busy adventure for the poop and pee."

7. I gave Wendy a Popsicle, but Melody rejected hers. Wendy scolded her. "It's good, girl."

8. Wendy explained to Melody, "Girls don't snore. If you snore that means you're a daddy."

9. Wendy asked me, "Mommy, do you think Kermit likes *The Muppet Show* or *Sesame Street* better?"

10. I overheard Wendy saying, "You know how we're in the same house but in different neighborhoods?"

11. She said to me, "You know what my favorite opposite is? The middle."

12. Wendy asked her sister, "Mooey, do you know what 'crowded' means? It means very, very crowded."

13. I overheard her say, "Yesterday is another word for last night."

14. She made up a song: "We're always together when we're with each other."

15. Wendy said, "When I look at food, I feel contagious."

16. She put a piece of Kleenex on her head and said, "Ahoy, matey!" Tim told me that once, in the car, she put a napkin on her head and said, "Mercy me!"

17. I asked her, "What's that on your finger?"
    She answered, "Nothing."
    She paused. "But it's not a booger."

18. Wendy asked, "Mommy, why did you marry daddy? Was it because we needed a dad?"

19. Wendy called Cruella DeVille *Cruella TeDilla*.

20. Wendy and Melody got sticks with horse heads to gallop around the house. When figuring out their names, Wendy said, "Mine is Sweet Lover."

21. She was pretending to talk on the phone. I heard her say, "That's all you got for me?"

22. We passed a landscaper's truck with leaves and branches sticking out. Wendy referred to it as the "salad truck."

23. She didn't like spaghetti sauce on her pasta. She told Tim, "I love clean noodles."

24. At Wendy's school, girls wear shorts under their dresses, so Wendy explained, "Yeah, it's a private school. We don't show our private parts."

25. She learned to write a little. She wrote something on a yellow Post-it and put it next to Bosco. The note said, *Cat are you.*

26. On the toilet, Wendy announced that she had peed and I said, "That's it?" She responded, "That was just a sizzle."

27. Melody asked Wendy, "How do you jump so high [off the swings]?" Wendy replied, "Well, I just use my talent, and . . . ."

28. Melody had a sock monkey with a red butt. Wendy knew that women who can have babies get their periods. So, Wendy looked at the monkey's red butt, and—very seriously—said, "The monkey is a girl. That's her blood."

29. We were taking a walk in our neighborhood—a faux New England neighborhood of small homes—and Melody was in a stroller. Wendy said, "I like walking with you." She paused. "We're two mommies." "Who's your baby?" I asked. She said, "Melody."

30. One time, I inadvertently put the garage door opener in my pocket, and every time I bent over, the door opened or closed. Of course, I had no clue why the door kept opening and closing (which is rather silly). My mom was at the house with us, and we were very alarmed: *Was someone in the garage? Were the doors locked? Maybe it was Tim, home at noon?* Both Wendy and Melody looked excitedly at the door into the garage, and Wendy declared, "It's Daddy!" My mom and I attempted to mask our anxiety about home invasion, and Wendy sensed it. She looked at me and calmly said, "It's OK, mommy. It's only a monster."

31. While in the car in line at the drive-thru at Burger King, Wendy said, "Mommy, Mooey has little nostrils. Her nostrils are cute."

Melody

1. I was changing Melody's diaper one day, but I kept her shoes on. Melody said that I was "doing it like grandma dooos it."

2. On bulldogs, Melody said, "They look cute, but they're actually ugly."

3. Melody, too, liked the cats—especially Jules. She said to me, "He's nice. Where you bought him?"

4. One morning, Melody heard Tim in the shower. She said, "Oh, Daddy. I love Daddy. Where you bought him?"

5. Hugging my legs, she asked, "Who bought this mommy?"

6. Melody would sometimes threaten us. When she wanted to be finished with dinner, she said, "If you don't let me be done, I won't button my pants."

7. On another time, she said, "If you don't give me a snack, I won't get dressed. . . . What's your choice?"

8. According to Melody, this is how a cat takes a bath: "He puts some licks on his paw."

9. Melody puked, and I told her not to touch Jules till she was cleaned up. She said, "We don't want to put him in the washer."
"No," I agreed. "Why do we not want to put Jules in the washer?"
"Because then he won't be soft anymore," she answered.

10. Melody declared, "I like how God made our kitty."

11. We passed a horse, and Melody said, "That's a big organic horse."

12. Melody asked, "When I'm in heaven, can I tell Jesus I wanna see my mommy?"

13. Melody had this habit of waking me up in the middle of the night for absurd requests, such as covering her with the blanket—which she could do herself. One night while I was pulling up her blanket, she noticed that Wendy's covers had been kicked off. She asked, "Will you cover my sister, too?"

14. The girls were supposed to clean up the mess they made in Tim's office. I asked, "How's daddy's office?"
Melody replied, "Clean as a feather."

15. Melody came across a photo from her first birthday at the Rainforest Café. She told me, "This is actually very special to me." She added, "Pack this when I go to heaven."

16. Melody wanted to go on the toilet like her sister. "I'm a big girl, mommy. I'm a big kid now," she said.

17. On the potty, she told me, "Help me go pee-pee, Momma. How I do it?" Sitting there, she said, "It doesn't work." She figured it out, and she told

Wendy, "Wendy, I have a pull-up on!" And then they both got M&M's whenever Melody got it right.

18. Melody said, "I don't like chickens because they're pointy."

19. Melody said to me, "You had three babies in your tummy."
    "I only had two," I told her.
    Melody protested, "I thought daddy was in your tummy."

20. At Boston Market, we were nearly done. Melody turned to Tim and asked, "What are we waiting for?"

21. While Tim was fixing a toilet, Melody looked at him and said, "What's the problem?"

22. When we were setting up Candyland, Melody put aside the instructions and said, "We don't need the recipe."

23. When Melody had a cold, she declared, "I'm just a sick little kid. I'm just a sick little girl."

24. She would hug me and say, "You're my best momma."

25. Melody would say, "I want Daddy to come home. I want Daddy to take care of me." She'd hug Wendy and say, "I love my sister."

26. While we were waiting for Wendy in her art class, Melody picked up a leaf and some man said to her, "That's your dinner."
    After the man left, Melody turned to me and said, "This isn't my dinner."

27. I was putting on makeup, and Melody was watching. She asked, "Can I have some lipstick?"
    "No," I answered.
    Melody offered her rebuttal, "I've been keeping my fingers out of my nose."

28. When I put three "Hello, Kitty" Band-Aids on her bug bites, she said, "I look beautiful."

29. We talked about things.
    "Did you burp?" I asked.
    "I burped twice."
    "What do you say?"
    "Excuse me. Excuse me."

30. Melody was looking at some rust on the gate at her school, and she declared that it was just spaghetti sauce.

31. When kissing Melody goodnight one night, I said, "Don't wake Mommy up."
    Melody replied, "Only if you have to pee or if you're hurt or if you need to draw something."

32. This was how Melody said goodbye to grandma: "Goodbye, sweet Grandma." We laughed when she said it, and Melody responded, "Can you get a picture of that?"

33. Melody called my bra my kneepads.

34. She said to her sister, "Wendy, I'm bored of this game. I wanna play go-see-Daddy."

35. When she had a tummy ache, she said, "Tomorrow, I'm only having one bessert."

36. Having learned about camouflage on "Sesame Street," Melody was looking for a stuffed animal, which happened to be under a blanket. She explained, "It was camouflaged."

37. Melody said, "My monkey has to go to the vet. He's always hanging on stuff."
    Wendy replied, "Oh, that's normal. Monkeys always do that."

38. Wendy said, "I smell cat puke."
    Melody responded, "No, that's just my breakfast."

Acknowledgments

So many people were supporting me during this cancer adventure. It seems impossible to acknowledge them all. I'm just going to be super general. Thank you to my dear friends, my mom (Marilynn Spiegel), Tracey Bublick, Ironwood Cancer and Research Centers (especially Dr. Rakesh Begai, Dr. Aaron Ambrad, and Kelsey) and the deluge of other medical professionals I met, Barbara with the bras, all of the moms and women—so many women—from church and school and Tim's work who gave us great food and invited my kids on play dates, old neighbors who knew the cancer ropes, the chemo nurses again and again, and Tim's awesome family. Also, I want to thank those who contributed to the writing process—by reading manuscripts, reading long-winded blog posts, pointing out writing and cancer resources, showing me the path to publication, and/or getting all serious about a memoir with me. A very special thank you to Karen Craigo for her keen editorial skills (she's been on board for three of my four books), and Wipf and Stock Publishers for including my mildly brazen work among their fine offerings.

Rest in Peace, Philando Castile.

I especially thank Tim, Wendy, and Melody over and over again. I love everything about you three.

About the Author

Jennifer Spiegel is the author of two novels, *And So We Die, Having First Slept* and *Love Slave*. She has also written the short story collection, *The Freak Chronicles*. Additionally, Spiegel is half of Snotty Literati, a book-reviewing duo with Lara Smith, and she works as an English professor. She lives in Phoenix with her family. For more information, please visit www.jenniferspiegel.com.

Made in the USA
Middletown, DE
29 January 2020